Clinical Atlas of
Sperm Morphology

Clinical Atlas of Sperm Morphology

AM Phadke
Consultant Andrologist
Ex. Hon. Executive Director
Family Welfare Bureau
Unit Family Planning Association of India
Mumbai, India

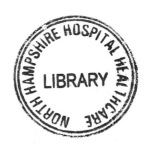

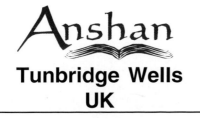

Tunbridge Wells
UK

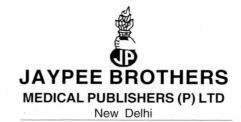

JAYPEE BROTHERS
MEDICAL PUBLISHERS (P) LTD
New Delhi

First published in the UK by

Anshan Ltd
in 2008
6 Newlands Road
Tunbridge Wells
Kent TN4 9AT, UK

Tel: +44 (0)1892 557767
Fax: +44 (0)1892 530358
E-mail: info@anshan.co.uk
www.anshan.co.uk

ISBN   978-1-905740-71-0

British Library Cataloguing in Publication Data
A catalogue record for this book is available from the British Library

Printed in India by Ajanta Offset & Packagings Ltd., New Delhi

To
My Wife
Manda

And my two sons
Dr. Avinash *and* **Dr. Dilip**
for their infinite patience,
loving forbearance and encouragement.

Foreword

Dr David Mortimer PhD
President
OOZOA Biomedical Inc., West Vancouver
Canada
Author of Practical Laboratory Andrology and
Formerly Scientific Director, Sydney IVF Centre
and a member of the advisory committee of World
Health Organization in the preparation of *3rd edition
of WHO Laboratory Manual for the examination Human
semen and sperm-cervical mucus interaction.*

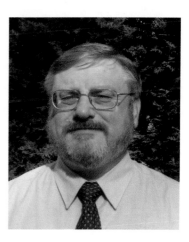

Human sperm morphology is a sensitive biomarker of a man's risk of fertility potential, as well as of his exposure to reproductive toxins. However, in this regard it is a negative indicator: an increased prevalence of atypical forms, and of their increasingly abnormality, indicates the likelihood of reduced fertility. But in order to understand the nature of abnormal human sperm morphology—especially when confronted with the legendary pleomorphism of the human spermatozoon — requires a deep understanding of the relationships between both sperm morphology and function, and sperm abnormalities and dysfunction. Careful examination of spermatozoa in stained smears is the fundamental tool employed in diagnostic andrology laboratories worldwide, yet many people look but do not see.

It is only in the past two years that I have come to know Dr Achyut Phadke, and I regret not having had the opportunity to have known him for far longer. His intense interest in sperm morphology is a pleasure to behold, especially in the days when researchers are busily pushing back the new frontiers of genomics, proteomics and metabolomics, for it is still working at the bench with a light microscope that the great majority of diagnoses of male factor infertility are made. Certainly this might change, but the careful assessment of sperm morphology from well-stained smears will not be displaced for many years yet. Therefore, we must continue to improve the educational materials available for training andrology laboratory scientists and technicians.

Dr Phadke's Clinical Atlas of Sperm Morphology represents the culmination of many years of tireless, patient effort by him, and will be a valuable educational resource for andrologists and spermatologists, not just in India, but around the world. As a result of this magnum opus at the culmination of his career I hope that he will take his place alongside other renowned workers in this field such as John MacLeod, Georges David, Rune Eliasson and, most recently, Roelof Menkveld and Thinus Kruger.

David Mortimer PhD
Vancouver, Canada

Preface

This Clinical Atlas of Sperm Morphology is not an erudite and scholarly monograph on the subject intended for the use of advanced research workers. Rather, it is an illustrated table guide, incorporating the basic concepts of sperm morphology, meant for beginners in the field of Andrology, technicians, postgraduate students, urologists, pathologists, gynecologists and laboratories associated with IVF and other assisted reproductive programs.

The relevant essential information about the subject of sperm morphology remains scattered in different books and articles in various scientific journals, and as such remains inaccessible to most clinicians. This treatise embodies the basic concepts of sperm morphology together with illustrative pictures to make it a comprehensive guide.

Keeping in mind the intended readership, this Atlas does not include Electron Microscopy or Trans Electron Microscopy pictures, which would be Greek and Latin to most of them.

I concede that the days of a book of single authorship are history. In the past, I have received persistent queries about various aspects of sperm morphology from the fellow clinicians, pathologists, urologists and gynecologists. These have provided the impetus for writing this book. I modestly submit that my vast experience of the last fifty two years as a practicing andrologist, semen analyst, pathologist and a research worker in the field of andrology sufficiently qualifies me to undertake the task of writing such an Atlas. Besides, there is no Atlas of Sperm morphology currently available.

Both of my sons are pathologists and from their comments and criticism I could understand the general expectations and viewpoint of pathologists.

A novel staining method using Rose Bengal and Toluidine Blue is used for the first time to illustrate the sperm morphology section. This method, invented by me, is based on the dye replacement technique. Similarly a modified Shorr's staining method is used to discriminate between the germinal and non-germinal cells. Likewise, the acrosomal lesions are dealt with in details.

How can I forget my mentors, well wishers, co-workers, teachers and guides who helped me during the development of my career? I would like to express my deepest gratitude to two enlightened women: Late Lady Dhanavanti Rama Rao and Late Mrs. Awabai Wadia (both ex-Presidents of the Family Planning Association of India and subsequently of the International Planned Parenthood Federation) for encouraging me and helping me financially from the meager resources that a NGO could have.

I sadly miss the presence of late Dr Mrs Shanta Rao PhD and late Dr Anil Seth PhD who were working in the then Institute For Research In Reproduction (ICMR) and with whom I had collaborated for more than a quarter of a century in carrying out my research work.

Late Dr GM Phadke FRCS, Ex- Hon. Director, Family Welfare Bureau (unit Family Planning Association of India) not only encouraged me in my research activities, but also had offered me a virtual carte blanche to incur financial expenses from funds that were at his disposal. With deep gratitude I pay my respects to his memories.

With heartfelt reverence I pay my respects to late Dr MC Chang who was my teacher and guide at the Worcester Foundation for Experimental Biology, Shrewsbury, Massachusetts, USA in 1963. Not only did he teach me the intricacies of reproductive physiology in laboratory animals, but also impressed on my mind the importance of being a good human being.

Dr Rune Eliasson and Dr David Mortimer have helped me by their comments and criticism from time to time.

I am deeply indebted to Dr David Mortimer, formerly Scientific Director Sydney IVF center and a member of the advisory committee of World Health Organization in the preparation of *3rd edition of WHO Laboratory Manual for the examination of Human semen and sperm-cervical mucus interaction,* for writing a foreword to this Atlas.

Likewise I express my thanks to Dr Kamala Gopalkrishnan, formerly of the then Institute for Research in Reproduction (ICMR) and a member of the advisory committee of World Health Organization in the preparation of *3rd edition of WHO Laboratory Manual for the examination of Human semen and sperm-cervical mucus interaction,* for meticulously going through the manuscript and making valuable suggestions

I also express my thanks to Jaypee Brothers Medical Publishers for undertaking to publish this book and bringing it out in such a beautiful form.

I must put on record that it was my elder son, Dr Avinash, without whose persistent insistence, repeated prodding and financial inputs for my research, this book would not have seen the light of the day.

Mumbai
India

Achyut M Phadke

Contents

Section 1

Clinical Atlas of Sperm Morphology

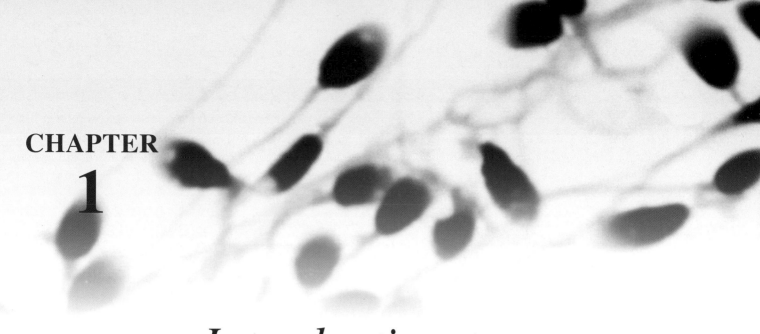

CHAPTER
1

Introduction to Sperm Morphology

DISCOVERY OF HUMAN SPERMATOZOA

Weisman (1941) has given an interesting and lucid account of discovery of spermatozoa. According to him in 1677, Antoj van Leeuwenhoek mentioned configuration of spermatozoa. In a famous letter written on 9th June 1699 to the Royal Society of London, he wrote, "I have discovered Animalcula in the masculine seed".

Dr Ham first saw spermatozoa under the microscope in August 1677. Subsequently, in March 1678, Nicholas Hartsoeker illustrated human spermatozoa for the first time.

French investigators give credit to this trio for having independently discovered human spermatozoa.

It is incredible that there was a long wait of more than two and half centuries for somebody to describe the acrosome. Williams (1934) described acrosome for the first time.

INTRODUCTION TO SPERM MORPHOLOGY

GENERAL CONSIDERATIONS

Assessment of sperm morphology is the most difficult aspect of semen analysis. It requires long experience and expertise on the part of the investigator. The subject of sperm morphology not only involves the study of morphology of normal and abnormal spermatozoa but also seeks to investigate the causal relationship between sperm abnormalities and infertility. The identification and characteristics of other cellular elements in semen, though by default is included in sperm morphology, is a separate subject and will be considered in a subsequent volume. The sperm morphology is a dynamic subject and has undergone periodic re-evaluation to keep pace with the ever-increasing scientific data.

There is unanimity amongst investigators regarding the role of certain isolated sperm abnormalities like spermatozoa with absence of acrosomes or tails and the presence of only "Pin headed" spermatozoa, as a causative factor in infertility. However, it is the relationship between the other sperm abnormalities and infertility, that remains as of now, a gray area beset with continuing debates and conflicting opinions. But it is hardly prudent to debunk this subject entirely on this basis.

NOMENCLATURE USED IN ANDROLOGY

Before starting the appraisal of sperm morphology, it is essential that the readers understand the different jargon words used by andrologists to express the sperm variables. Eliason (1970), Mortimer (1994) and WHO manual (1999) provide the requisite explanation of the different terms used by andrologists. Note that the term "spermia" refers to the volume of the ejaculate and "zoospermia" refers to the number of spermatozoa in the ejaculate.

Table 1.1 explains the nomenclature used in andrology.

Table 1.1: Nomenclature used in andrology	
1. Aspermia	Absence of the ejaculate.
2. Azoospermia	Absence of spermatozoa in the ejaculate.
3. Hypospermia	Abnormally low volume of the ejaculate.
4. Hyperspermia	Abnormally high volume of the ejaculate.
5. Normozoospermia	Normal ejaculate as per WHO standards (1999)
6. Oligozoospermia: (severe)	Sperm concentration $< 10 \times 10^6$ /ml.
(mild)	Sperm concentration between 10×10^6 /ml to 20×10^6 /ml.
7. Asthenozoospermia	(a) Less than 50% spermatozoa with rapid progressive motility and slow sluggish motility. Or (b) Less than 25% spermatozoa with rapid progressive activity or decreased sperm motility (Usually < 40%)
8. Teratozoospermia	Increased number of spermatozoa with abnormal morphology. (Typically > 50% abnormal forms)
9. Oligoasthenoteratozoospermia	Signifies disturbance of all the three parameters.
10. Necrozoospermia	All the spermatozoa in the ejaculate are dead as confirmed by vital staining.
11. Polyzoospermia	Means a very high concentration of spermatozoa in the ejaculate. (e.g. 250×10^6/ml)
12. Bacteriospermia	Presence of large number of bacteria in the semen.
13. Pyospermia	Presence of large number of leukocytes in the semen.
14. Hemospermia	Presence of blood in semen.

CHARACTERISTICS AND IMPORTANCE OF SPERM MORPHOLOGY

The volume, sperm count and sperm motility are variable parameters of ejaculates in infertile and fertile men and are influenced by various physiological and pathological factors enumerated below.

Physiological factors	Pathological factors
• Age	• Systemic and local infection
• Period of abstinence	• Systemic diseases like diabetes and anemia
• Method of collection	• Drugs: Nitrofurans, antidepressants, excess of vitamin A
• Inadequate ejaculations	• Associated hernia, hydrocele and varicocele
• Increased body or scrotal temperatures	• Filariasis
• Climatic conditions	• Anxiety and stress
• Personal habits like consumption of alcohol and smoking	

RELATIVELY STABLE PARAMETER

Comparatively, sperm morphology is considered a relatively stable parameter in the ejaculate. Even then infection, trauma, other testicular stress situations, certain drugs and hormones influence it. (McLeod 1956, 1966, 1970): David et al., (1972).

REFLECTS A COMPREHENSIVE PICTURE OF EVENTS OCCURRING IN THE TESTIS AND EPIDIDYMIS

Testicular Factors

Leydig cells dysfunction: Sperm abnormalities are genetically determined (Wyrobeck and Bruce 1978). The first mechanism operates at the level of spermatogonia/spermatocytes, which is influenced by abnormal Leydig cell function. This will result in abnormal acrosomal development.

Sertoli cell dysfunction: The Sertoli cells are susceptible to the environmental factors and stress. The disturbed Sertoli cell function adversely affects spermiogenesis and results in the production of simple reversible elongation of sperm head. The severe elongation of sperm head is irreversible.

The genesis of the other sperm abnormalities is discussed in the narrations of the individual entities.

Epididymal Factors

When a spermatid is released from a Sertoli cell during spermiogenesis, a cytoplasmic tag remains attached to it. This cytoplasmic tag is divided into two unequal parts. The larger tag separates gradually from the sperm cell and forms the residual body. During the sperm maturation in the epididymis, the smaller cytoplasmic tag remaining attached to the sperm cell is gradually lost. The presence of large number of spermatozoa in the ejaculate with attached cytoplasmic droplets–denoting their immaturity–is indicative of epididymal dysfunction.

SELECTION OF PHYSIOLOGICALLY MATURE SPERMATOZOA

The description of physiologically normal spermatozoa is based on the studies of twin physiological conditions; the post coital sperm migration and binding of spermatozoa to zona pellucida during fertilization in "in vivo and in vitro" situations.

POST COITAL SPERM MIGRATION

Mortimer et al., (1982) and Fredricsson and Bjork (1977), in the post coital tests, studied the sperm populations in the cervical mucus at the level of internal os and at the level of the external os. These observers noted that during the post coital process, there was significantly higher percentage of abnormal sperms present in the cervical mucus at the level of external os than at the level of internal os. The healthy cervical mucus seemed to possess a mysterious ability of denying access to the abnormal sperms (excepting microsperms and elongated sperms) into the cervical canal. Hence, barring these two sperm abnormalities, spermatozoa recovered from the endocervical mucus in the post coital tests represented functionally normal spermatozoa. However, Menkveld was the first investigator to advocate the concept of taking these spermatozoa as a referral standard for 'normal' spermatozoa (1987).

BINDING OF SPERMATOZOA TO THE ZONA PELLUCIDA DURING FERTILIZATION

Menkveld et al., (1991) carried out studies, in vitro, regarding the morphology of spermatozoa found tightly bound to the zona pellucida, as seen in hemizona assays. Liu and Baker (1992) on the other hand carried out studies "in vivo", regarding the morphology of spermatozoa found tightly bound to zona pellucida during fertilization.

The characteristics of 'normal' spermatozoa found bound to zona pellucida, both in 'in vivo' as well as in 'in vitro' conditions were akin to the characteristics of 'normal' spermatozoa recovered from post coital endocervical mucus.

MORPHOLOGICAL CHARACTERISTICS OF NORMAL SPERMATOZOA

Human spermatozoa belong to a select group of species in whom there is marked heterogeneity of spermatozoa in semen. This is in contrast with the situation in other species, including subhuman primates, where there is uniformity of form and structure of spermatozoa (Zamboni et al., 1971).

WHO CRITERIA

An ideal method for studying normal spermatozoa would be to study in in vivo condition, the morphological characteristics of those spermatozoa that are engaged in ovum penetration. As this is not possible in humans, an alternative model has to be relied upon. Hence the physiologically normal spermatozoa, present in the endocervical mucus at the level of internal os in the post coital process, are taken as representative of normal forms. Papanicolaou-stained endocervical normal sperm population, despite some inevitable shrinkage, is used for studying the morphological characteristics of normal forms.

There are dual reasons as to why the so-called 'Normal' spermatozoa observed in the semen of fertile men cannot be relied upon to serve as a referral standard, firstly because in the semen smears a homogenous sperm population of normal spermatozoa is seldom available for studying their morphological characteristics and secondly the physiological status of such normal forms remains unproven.

TYGERBERG STRICT CRITERIA

Strict criteria for sperm morphology, originally described by Kruger et al., (1986) were based on the data obtained from IVF results. These authors observed that there were no pregnancies where the semen samples contained < 14% normal forms but the overall pregnancy rate was 25.8% where the semen samples contained > 14% normal forms.

However in the next year Kruger et al., (1987) reported that a fertilization rate of 49.4% per oocyte was noted where the semen samples contained <14% normal forms. With the semen samples having > 14% normal forms an overall fertilization rate of 88.3% per oocyte was achieved.

Method of Study

The stained slide is examined under an oil immersion (1000 x) with a light microscope and an ocular micrometer, calibrated with a stage micrometer, is used for the exact morphometric measurements.

Table 1.2 Summarizes the criteria of morphologically normal spermatozoa as per "strict" criteria and WHO criteria.

Table 1.2: Criteria for morphologically normal spermatozoa		
Papanicolaou stain	*Strict criteria (1991)*	*WHO criteria (1999)* *Sperm head, neck, midpiece and tail should be normal.*
Head	Smooth oval configuration	Oval with regular smooth outline. A slightly different shape, recognized as normal, is oval in shape but is slightly tapered at the post acrosomal end.
Acrosome	Acrosome should comprise about 40 to 70% of anterior sperm head.	Acrosomal area should comprise 40 to 70% of the head area.
Head length	3-5 μm	4-5 μm
Head width	2-3 μm Head width should be between three-fifth and two-thirds of the normal head length.	2.5 – 3.5 μm The length to width ratio should be 1.5 to 1.75
Borderline normal head forms	Regarded as abnormal.	Considered abnormal.
Presence of vacuole **Micrometric measurements**		Presence of solitary vacuole considered normal. Necessary.
Neck	No abaxial implantation and must be normal.	
Midpiece	Slender (axially attached). Approximately 1 μm in width and approximately 1 ½ times the head length. No cytoplasmic droplets of more that half the head size.	Slender, less that 1μm in width and about 1½ times the length of the head. Attached centrally to the head. The cytoplasmic droplets should be less than half the size of sperm head.
Tail	Uniform, slightly thinner than the midpiece, uncoiled, approximately 45 μm long.	Uniform, straight, thinner than the midpiece and un coiled. It should be approximately 45 μm in length.

INDIVIDUALISM IN THE SEMEN PICTURES OF INFERTILE MEN

The morphological characteristics of semen show marked variations in different individuals, but there is a relative constancy of the same in a given individual, so much so, that it has been stated that his semen may identify a man. Thus Moench (1934) stated that the sperm morphology serves as a means of identifying an individual and repeated his claim in 1952. Joel and Pollack (1940) substantiated Moench's claim and added that such identification may have forensic value. MacLeod (1962) even stated that the cytology of the ejaculate might be considered analogous to the fingerprint of that individual.

However, this relative constancy of the morphological features in semen of any man may alter suddenly in response to toxic chemical substances, increased exposure to heat, and during an episode of chickenpox and pneumonia or following severe allergic reactions.

SPERM MORPHOLOGY AND NATURAL FERTILIZATION

Moench and Holt (1932) had claimed that the morphology of sperm head seems to be the most reliable indicator of fertilizing power of the cells.

However, several investigators have stated that sperm morphology played little or no role in natural fertilization (Singer et al., (1980), Aitken et al., (1982), Zaini et al., (1985) and Van Zyl et al., (1990)).

Nevertheless, Van Zyl et al., (1990) have also stated that there are poor chances of in vivo fertilization if the percentage of normal forms is less than 4%.

THE STUDY OF SPERM MORPHOLOGY

The study of sperm morphology has undergone successive evolutionary stages regarding its aims and methodology.

ERA OF RECORDING OF SPERM ABNORMALITIES

Maddox (1984) described the abnormalities of spermatozoa for the first time. Martin et al., (1902) not only illustrated abnormal spermatozoa but also described measurements of different parts taken with the aid of screw micrometer. Carry (1916) summarized the literature to that date.

CORRELATION BETWEEN SPERM MORPHOLOGY AND INFERTILITY

Percentage of Abnormal Sperms in Fertile and Infertile Men

Initially the investigators strived to find out the relationship between sperm morphology and infertility on the basis of the incidence of abnormal spermatozoa present in the semen of fertile and infertile men. Three representative studies are considered here. Thus Hotchkiss (1944) noted that the incidence of abnormal sperms was 15.8% in the semen of 105 infertile men as against 10.9% in the semen of 200 fertile men.

Aitken et al., (1982) studied a selected group of unexplained infertile couples, in which the sperm concentration and motility were within normal range and concluded that increased percentage of abnormal sperms was possibly the etiological factor.

MacLeod and Gold (1952) carried out an exhaustive comparative study, based on the detailed statistical data, of the semen quality in 1000 men of known fertility and 800 cases of infertile marriages. Regarding the sperm morphology in these two groups the authors observed that abnormalities in morphology increased with decreasing sperm counts and they were more frequently found in infertile men with low sperm counts.

Investigators soon realized that it was futile to attempt to establish correlation between the sperm abnormalities and infertility for several reasons. The criteria as to what constitutes a 'normal' sperm were not standardized and each laboratory had its own norms in this regards. Several other vexing questions also remained unanswered. Out of several abnormal forms, which were to be identified for such a comparative study? How the question of multiple sperm abnormalities was to be resolved? Were the concerned abnormal forms viable and motile? What were the permissible limits of sperm abnormalities in cases of known fertility?

In the reference values of fertility potential WHO manual (1999) has refrained from stating any percentage of normal and abnormal forms pending the results of   multicentric population based studies that are now in progress.

The most important drawback of such studies was that no cognizance was taken of normal physiological post coital processes.

Thus one is reminded of Hunner (1921) who wrote, "If there are many actively moving spermatozoa present, per microscopic field, sperm morphology is of no importance and the presence of many abnormal spermatozoa will have no influence on the outcome of the post-coital process."

While endorsing the opinion of Hunner, Cary and Hotchkiss (1934) had stated "Abnormal forms may possess motility, but are rarely if ever, found in the upper layer of the cervical mucus in the post-coital process and we must consider them ineffectual in fertilization."

These difficulties forced the investigators to focus their attention on 'normal', rather than 'abnormal', forms for carrying out the comparative studies of semen of 'fertile' and 'infertile' populations.

The Incidence of Sperms with Normal Morphology in the Semen of Fertile and Infertile Men

Glezarman and Batoov (1993) reported that in the fertile semen samples the percentage of normal forms varied in the range of 4 to 45%. Haidl and Schill (1993) found a mean of 29.5% normal spermatozoa in fertile population with Düsseldorf criteria. On the other hand Menkveld et al., (1990) noted a mean of 16.7% normal spermatozoa in infertile population using strict Tygerberg criteria.

Similarly, reduced fertility and longer interval to first pregnancy was found to be associated with reduced percentage of normal forms (Bartoov et al., 1982; Bostole et al., 1982).

Likewise higher percentage of sperms with normal morphology was found in fertile semen donors in A.I.D. programs (Edwinson et al. 1983: McGoven et al., 1983).

However, Zaini et al., (1985) and Polansky and Lamb (1988) found no predictive value in sperm morphology, as well as other semen parameters, on the existence of male infertility.

Data Obtained from Intrauterine Inseminations

In intrauterine inseminations with oligozoospermic and asthenozoospermic semen, there was a correlation between the percentage of normal forms and pregnancy rate (Francavilla et al., 1990).

Inputs Received from IVF Results

Tygerberg hospital IVF results were reported by Kruger et al., (1986). With greater than 15% morphologically normal spermatozoa, the fertilization rate was 82.5% with a pregnancy incidence of 25.6%. When the percentage of normal spermatozoa was less than 14%, the fertilization rate dropped drastically to 37% and no pregnancies were recorded.

In Norfolf IVF center, Oehninger et al., (1988) reported the data regarding sperm morphology and pregnancy successes. These authors reported the pregnancy rate of 32% where the percentage of normal sperms was > 14%; the pregnancy rate of 25% where the percentage of normal sperms ranged between 4 – 14% and the pregnancy rate of only 7% where the percentage of normal forms was < 4%.

WHO manual (1999) has summed up the current situation as follows: "Data from assisted reproductive technology programs suggest that, as the percentage of sperm morphology falls below 15% normal forms, using the methods and definitions described in this manual, the rate of fertilization in 'in vitro' decreases."

SPERM MORPHOLOGY AND ACCIDENTS OF PREGNANCIES

Several investigators sought to investigate if there was any relationship between sperm morphology and accidents of pregnancy like miscarriages, ectopic pregnancies and stillbirths. Bender, S. (1952), Swyer (1953), Joel (1955), MacLeod and Gold (1957), and Hartman (1965), concluded that there was no relation between the poor sperm morphology and accidents of pregnancy.

BIBLIOGRAPHY

1. Aitken RJ, Best, FSM, Richardson, DW, et al. An analysis of sperm function in case of unexplained infertility: Conventional criteria, movement characteristics and fertilizing capacity. Fertil Steril 1982; 30: 212.
2. Bartoov B, Eites F, Langsam J, Synder M, Fisher J. Ultrastructural studies in morphological assessment of human spermatozoa. Int J Androl 1982; 5: 81.
3. Bender S. The end results of primary sterility. Brit Med J 1952; 2: 409.
4. Bostole E, Serup J, Raffe H. Relation between morphologically abnormal spermatozoa and pregnancies obtained during a 20 year follow up period. Int J Androl 1982; 5: 379.
5. Cary HW. Examination of semen with reference to gynecological aspects. Am. J. Obstet. Dis women child 1916; 74: 615.
6. Carry WH, Hotchkiss RS. Sperm appraisal, A differential stain that advances the study of sperm morphology. J Am Med Assos 1934; 102: 587.
7. David G, Bisson JP, Jouannet, et al. Les teratospermies. In Thiboult C (Ed.) La sterilitie due male. Aquisions recents. Masson et cie, Paris, 1972.
8. Edwinson A, Bergman P, Steen Y, Nilsson S. Characteristics of donor semen and cervical mucus at the time of conception. Fertil Steril 1983; 30: 327.
9. Francavilla, Romano R, Santucci R, Poccia G. Effects of sperm morphology and motile sperm count on outcome of intrauterine insemination in oligozoospermia and/or asthenozoospermia Fertil Steril 1990; 53: 892.
10. Eliasson R, Hellinga G, Luebcke F, et al. Empfehlungen zur Bomenklatur in der Andrlogie. Androllegia, 1970; 2: 186.
11. Eliason R. Standards for investigation for human semen. Andrologie 1971; 3: 49.
12. Fredricson B, Bjork R. Morphology of post-coital spermatozoa in cervical secretions and its clinical significance. Fertil Steril 1977; 28: 841.
13. Glezerman, Marek, Bartoov Benjamin. Semen analysis in Infertility Male and Female. (ed,) Insler, VS and Luenfield, B Churchill Livingstone, London 1993; 295.
14. Haidl G, Schill WB. Sperm morphology in fertile men. Arch Androl 1993; 31: 153.
15. Hartman CG. Correlation among criteria of semen quality. Fertil Steril 1965; 16: 662.
16. Hotchkiss RS. Fertility in men. William Hieneman (Medical Books) Limited. London. 1944; 130.
17. Huhner M. Methods for examining spermatozoa in the diagnosis and treatment of sterility. Int J Surg 1921; 34: 91.
18. Joël CA. The role of spermatozoa in habitual abortion. Fertil Steril 1955; 6: 459.
19. Joël K, Pollak OJ. Die Spermaauntersuchung nach dem heutigen Stander Forschung. Helvet Med Acta 1940; 7: 70.
20. Kruger TF, Menkveld R, Stander FSH et al. Sperm morphology features as a prognostic factor in in vitro fertilization. Fertil Steril 1986; 44: 118.
21. Kruger TF, Acosta AA, Simmons KF, Swanson RJ, Matla JF, Oehminger S. Predictive value of abnormal sperm morphology in in vitro fertilization. Fertil Steril 1988; 49: 112.
22. Kruger TF, Acosta AA, Simmons KE, Swanson RJ, Matta JF, Veek LL, Morshedi M, Burgo S. Urology 1987; 30:(3):248.
23. Liu DY, Baker HWG. Morphology of spermatozoa bound to the zona pellucida of human oocytes that failed to fertilize in vitro. J Reprod Fertil 1992; 94: 71.
24. Mc Gowan MP, Baker MWG, Kosias GT, Rennie G. Selection of high fertility donors for artificial insemination programmes. Clin Reprod Fertil 1983; 2: 269.
25. MacLeod J. Human semen. (Current Reviews) Fertil. Steril, 1956; 7: 368.
26. MacLeod J. A possible factor in the etiology of human fertility: Preliminary report. Fertil Steril 1962; 13: 29.
27. MacLeod J. The clinical implications of deviations in human spermatogenesis as evidenced in seminal cytology and experimental production of these deviations. Ex Med Int Cong Ser No. 133 P563, Proceedings of the Fifth Congress on Fertility and Sterility, Stockholm, 1966; 16-22.
28. Macleod J. The significance of deviation in human sperm morphology in human testis. Adv Exp Med Biol 1970; 10: 481.
29. Macleod J, Gold RZ. The male factor in fertility and infertility, IV Sperm morphology in fertile and infertile marriage. Fertil Steril 1952; 2: 394.
30. MacLeod J, Gold RJ. The male factor in fertility and infertility. IX Semen quality in relation to accidents of pregnancy. Fertil Steril 1957; 8: 36.
31. Maddox RL. Alquras observaciones sobre varias formas del espermatozoo de Cadez, Gac Med de cadez 1894; 11: 252.
32. Martin E, Carhett JS, Levi MF, Pennington MF. Study of morphology of human spermatozoa, Univ Penn Med Bull 1902; 2:15.

33. Menkveld R. An investigation of environmental influences on spermatogenesis and semen parameters. PhD. Dissertation Faculty of Medicine, University of Stellenbosch, South Africa 1987.

34. Menkveld R, Stander FSH, Kotz TJ vW, Kruger TF, Van Zyl JA. The evaluation of morphological characteristics of human spermatozoa according to stricter criteria. Human Reprod 1990; 5: 586.

35. Menkveld R. Appendices in Menkveld R, Oettle EE, Kruger TF, Swanson RJ, Oehninger S (eds.) Atlas of Human Sperm Morphology. p. 115. Williams and Wilkins. Baltimore 1991.

36. Menkveld R, Kruger TF, Oettle EE, Swanson RJ, Oehninger RJ, Oehninger S. (eds) Atlas of human sperm morphology, p 1. Williams and Wilkins. Baltimore 1991.

37. Moench GL, Holt H. Biometric studies of head lengths of human spermatozoa. J Lab Clin Med 1932; 17: 297.

38. Moench GL. Sperm morphology and biometrics as a means of identification of the individual. M. Times, New York 1934; 62:33.

39. Moench GL. Männliche Fruchtbarkeit In Biologie and Pathologie des Weibes (ed 2), L Seitz, (Ed). Berlin, 1952; 476.

40. Mortimer D, Leslie EE, Kelley RW and Templeton AA. Morphological selection of human spermatozoa in Vivo and in Vitro. J Reprod Fertil 1982; 64: 391.

41. Mortimer D. Practical laboratory Andrology. P.25 (Oxford University Press) Oxford, 1994.

42. Oehninger S, Acosta AA, Kruger TF, Veeck LL, Flood J, Jones HW. Failure of fertilization in in vitro fertilization: "Occult" male factor. J. In Vitro Fertil Embryo Transfer 1988; 5: 181.

43. Polansky FF, Lamb EJ. Do the results of semen analysis predict future fertility? A survival analysis study. Fertil Steril 1988; 49: 1059.

44. Singer R, Sagiv M, Barnet M, Segercich E, Allalaiouf F, Landav B, Servadio C. Motility, viability and percentage of morphologically abnormal forms of human spermatozoa in relation to sperm counts. Andrologia 1980; 12: 92.

45. Swyer GIM. Discussion of male infertility. Proc R Soc Med 1953; 46: 835.

46. Van Zyl JA, Kotze TJvW and Menkveld R. Predictive value of spermatozoa morphology in natural fertilization. In Acosta, A. A., Swanson RJ, Ackerman SN, Krger TF, Van Zyl JA, Menkveld R. (eds): Human Spermatozoa in Assisted Reproduction. P.319. Williams and Wilkins, Baltimore 1990.

47. Weisman, Abner I. Spermatozoa and sterility. Paul B Hoeber Inc Medical book department of Harper Brothers. New York. 1941; 1-2.

48. Williams WW. Spermatic abnormalities. New Eng J Med 1937; 217: 946.

49. Williams WW, Mac Guigan A, Carpenter HD. The staining and morphology of human spermatozoa. J Urol 1934; 32: 201.

50. World Health Organization. WHO Laboratory manual for the examination of human semen and sperm-cervical mucus interaction. 4th edn. (Cambridge: Cambridge University Press), 1999.

51. Wyrobeck AJ, Bruce WR. Induction of sperm shape abnormalities in mice and humans. In Hollandare, A, de-Serres, FJ. (eds) Chemical mutagens. Volume 5. Plenum, New York, 1978.

52. Zaini A, Jennings NG, Baker MWG. Are conventional sperm morphology and motility assessments of predictive value in subfertile men? Int. J Androl 1985; 8:427.

53. Zamoboni L, Rabbe H, Hamman R. The fine structure of monkey and human spermatozoa. Analyt Rec 1971; 169: 129.

54. Zaneveld LJD, Polakashi KL. Collection and physical examination of the ejaculate. In Hafez ESE (ed): Techniques of Human Andrology. Elsevier/North Holland, Amsterdam 1977; 147.

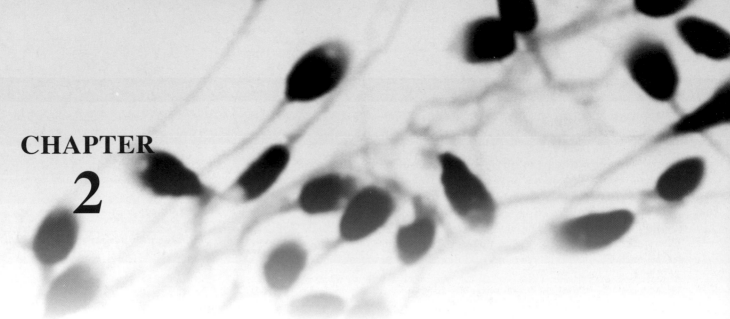

CHAPTER
2

Morphology of Human Spermatozoon

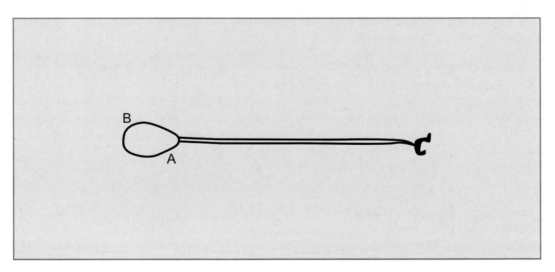

(The first known representation of human spermatozoon, after Hartsoekar 1678)

Adapted and modified from Weisman (1941). Spermatozoa And Sterility. Paul B. Hoeber, Inc. Medical book department of Harper & Brothers. London.

MORPHOLOGY OF HUMAN SPERMATOZOON

Many of the structures illustrated in the following figures are not visible by light microscope and the minute detailed information provided by electron microscopy and electron transmission microscopy is incorporated in these figures. This will enable the reader to have the basic knowledge of the structure of human sperm.

The spermatozoon is a specialized cell and differs from other body cells. The total length of a sperm is about 60 μm equal to that of the nucleus of ovum (Chatterjee CC, 2003). It has a *head, neck (or the connecting piece)* and *tail.* The tail has three constituent parts, namely, the *middle piece,* the *principal piece* and the *end piece.* The dimensions of the constituent parts of the spermatozoon are summarized below (Mortimer, D. 1994).

	Length	Width	Thickness
Head	3.0 – 5.0 µm	2.0 – 3.0 µm	Maximum 1.5 µm
Neck	0.3 µm		
Tail			
Middle piece	3.0 – 5.0 µm	1.0 µm	
Principal piece	40 – 50 µm	0.5 µm	
End piece	4.0 – 6.0 µm		

HEAD (FIGURES 2.1A AND B)

The sperm head is a plate like elastic structure, ovoid in shape, slightly tapered anteriorly. The thickness of the sperm head gradually increases from the apex towards the base so that it is seen as oval in shape when viewed from the front but appears to be pointed, like a spearhead, when viewed from the side. The head consists of an oval nucleus that is slightly tapered towards the apex and has a shallow recess in the base called *implantation fossa.* The nucleus is surrounded by a *nuclear membrane.* A double-layered acrosomal cap covers anteriorly about 30 to 70% of the nuclear area. The *outer acrosomal membrane* is just inside the plasma membrane while the inner *acrosomal membrane* is in immediate proximity of the nuclear membrane.

In between the inner and the outer acrosomal membranes lies the acrosomal matrix. A *posterior nuclear cap* covers the post-acrosomal portion of the nucleus. Externally a delicate plasma membrane envelops the head. The sperm head has very little cytoplasm. Thus, the sperm head is divided into two unequal parts, acrosomal and post-acrosomal regions, by a furrow that completely encircles the head.

The Nuclear Characteristics

1. The nucleus consists of extremely condensed chromatin and therefore appears to have a homogenous appearance even when examined by electron microscope. (Gray's Anatomy 1996). Defects in condensation of the nuclear material are often visible under light microscope as relatively clear areas or *nuclear vacuoles.* The extreme condensation of nuclear chromatin makes the sperm head highly resistant to various physical stresses. The other important nuclear characteristics that are summarized by Chatterjee (2003) are as follows:
2. The nucleus consists of 40% DNA.
3. It is rich in Arginine.
4. It has a strong affinity for basic dyes.
5. It absorbs ultraviolet rays.
6. It is refractory to deoxyribonuclease.

NECK (FIGURES 2.1 A AND B)

The *neck* is also called the *connecting piece* because it ensures intimate union between the head and tail of spermatozoon. The plasma membrane that surrounds the head continues to surround the neck and the tail of spermatozoon. The neck contains remnants of posterior nuclear cap and some cytoplasm. There are two

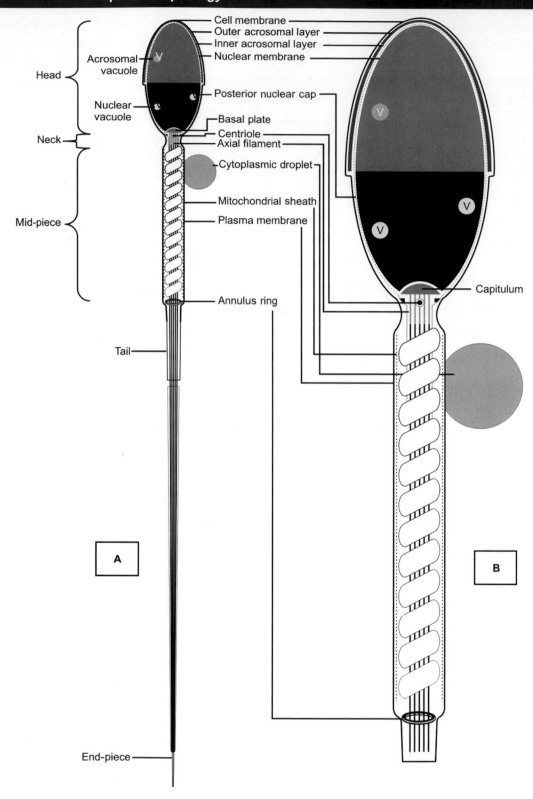

Head

Acrosomal vacuole

Nuclear vacuole

Neck

Mid-piece

Tail

End-piece

Cell membrane
Outer acrosomal layer
Inner acrosomal layer
Nuclear membrane

Posterior nuclear cap

Basal plate
Centriole
Axial filament
Cytoplasmic droplet

Mitochondrial sheath
Plasma membrane

Annulus ring

Capitulum

A

B

Figures 2.1A and B: Schematic drawing of human sperm

important structures seen in the neck, namely, the *basal body* and the *proximal centriole*. Proximally the *neck* is connected to the nuclear basal plate. Distally it is connected to the *middle piece.*

The *basal body* in its proximal part has a plate like fibrous structure, called *capitulum,* which fits into the depression (*implantation fossa*) in the base of the nucleus. In addition, nine, segmented-rod like structures, are seen in the neck region. Each of this segmented-rod like structure is continuous distally with the corresponding coarse fibril of the *axial filament.* The *proximal centriole* comes to lie just below the *implantation fossa.* The *axial filament* begins just behind the proximal centriole from the *posterior end knob* that originates from the distal centriole of spermatid. It passes through the *middle piece* and extends into the tail. At the junction of the middle piece and the principal piece the axial filament passes through a ring like structure called the *annulus.*

MIDDLE PIECE (FIGURES 2.1B AND 2.2 A)

It is a long cylindrical structure consisting of the central *axial filament* surrounded by the *mitochondrial sheath* and is enveloped by the cell membrane. In the *mitochondrial sheath* the mitochondria of the spermatid are arranged in a helical (spiral) manner. In humans there are twelve turns of mitochondrial helix (Mann, T. 1964). The mitochondrial sheath provides the sperm with energy for motility.

The *axial filament* is comprised of a *fibrous sheath,* which surrounds several longitudinal fibrils in a particular manner. The *fibrous sheath* is composed of several branching and interlinking semicircular strands or *ribs* held together by their attachment to two *longitudinal bars* located at opposite sides. These longitudinal bars run along the tail.

Immediately inside the fibrous sheath is a layer of *nine coarse fibrils.* These fibrils are petal shaped and are of unequal size and are present in the middle piece and the principal piece of the tail but are absent in the end piece.

Inside the layer of nine coarse fibrils is a *layer of nine pairs of doublets of microtubules.* Each pair of doublet of microtubule is situated on the inner side each coarse fibril.

Finally the core of the axial bundle consisting of *a central pair of microtubules* is present inside of the nine pair of doublets of microtubules. There are *radial links* from the coarse fibrils to the central pair of microtubules.

PRINCIPAL PIECE (FIGURE 2.2B)

This is the motile part of the tail and forms the greater part of the tail. It provides most of the propellant machinery to the sperm (Kruger TF, Menkveld R and Oehninger S 1996).

The structure of the principal piece is akin to that of the middle piece that is divested of its mitochondrial sheath. The coarse nine fibrils of the middle piece progressively diminish in thickness and finally disappear leaving only the inner fibrils in the axial core for much of the length of the principal piece.

As mentioned earlier, inside the layer of fibrous sheath are *nine coarse fibrils* with numbers designated from 1 to 9 in a clockwise manner. The line joining fibril 3 and 8 divides the tail into a *major compartment* containing 4 fibrils and a *minor compartment* containing 3 fibrils. This line also passes through both of the central microtubules and provides an axis in reference of which sperm movements can be analyzed (Inderbir Singh & Pal, G.A.2003).

END PIECE (FIGURE 2.2C)

The end-piece consists of the central pair of microtubules surrounded by the plasma membrane.

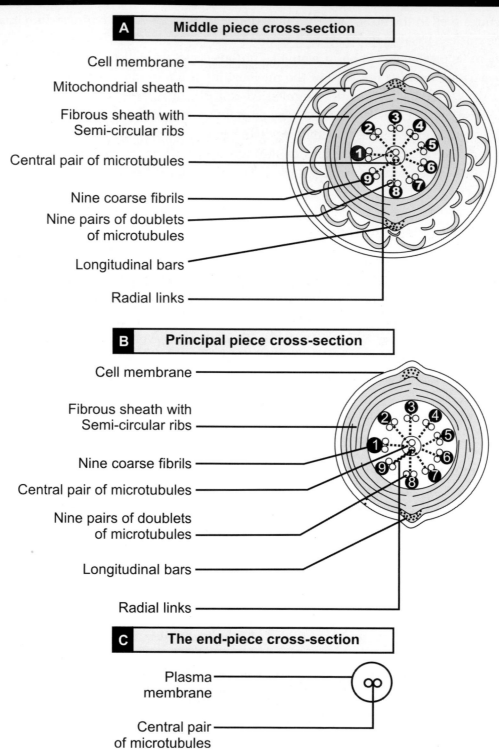

A **Middle piece cross-section**

Cell membrane

Mitochondrial sheath

Fibrous sheath with
Semi-circular ribs

Central pair of microtubules

Nine coarse fibrils

Nine pairs of doublets
of microtubules

Longitudinal bars

Radial links

B **Principal piece cross-section**

Cell membrane

Fibrous sheath with
Semi-circular ribs

Nine coarse fibrils

Central pair of microtubules

Nine pairs of doublets
of microtubules

Longitudinal bars

Radial links

C **The end-piece cross-section**

Plasma
membrane

Central pair
of microtubules

Figures 2.2A to C: Morphology of sperm tail (highly diagrammatic)

Proximal Centriole and Axis Filament (Figure 2.3)

The origin of the proximal centriole and the axial filament is better understood by following the development of a spermatid. In the earlier stage a pair of centrioles, which lie at right angles to each other, is close to the Golgi complex on the top of the nucleus. During the *Cap phase* these centrioles migrate to the opposite pole of the nucleus in the region of the *implantation fossa.* The centriole that is parallel to the long axis is called the *distal centriole* and constitutes the *basal body.* The centriole that is at right angles to the long axis remains unchanged and lodges itself in the neck region just below the *capitulum* in the *implantation fossa* (Gray's Anatomy 1996).

TRANSFORMATION OF SPERMATID
A Highly Schematic Drawing Modified after
Inderbeer Singh and Pal GB (2003)

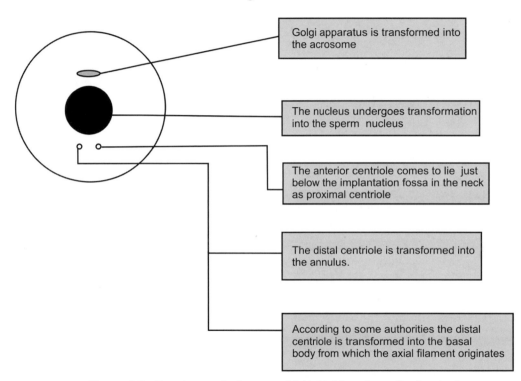

Golgi apparatus is transformed into the acrosome

The nucleus undergoes transformation into the sperm nucleus

The anterior centriole comes to lie just below the implantation fossa in the neck as proximal centriole

The distal centriole is transformed into the annulus.

According to some authorities the distal centriole is transformed into the basal body from which the axial filament originates

Figure 2.3: Development of spermatid (A highly schematic drawing)
Adapted from Inderbeer Singh and Paul, GB (2003)

BIBLIOGRAPHY

1. Chatterjee CC. Human Physiology 10th Edition. Medical Allied Agency, Kolkatta, 2003; 215-26.
2. Gray's Anatomy. 38th Edition (eds). Late Peter L. William, Banister, Lawrence, W, Berry, Martin, H, Collins, Patricia, Dyson, Mary, Dussek, Julian E, Fergusson, Mark WJ. Churchill Livingstone, London 1996.
3. Inderbir Singh, Pal GB. Human Embryology 10th Edition. Macmillan India Limited, Mumbai, 2003; 15-17.
4. Kruger TF, Menkveld R, Oehninger S. Anatomy of mature spermatozoa in Assisted Reproduction (eds). Acosta, AA and Kruger, TF Parthenon Publishing group London, 1996; 13-17.
5. Mann T. Biochemisrey of semen and of the male reproductive tract. Methuen and Company London, 1964; 26.
6. Mortimer D. Practical laboratory Andrology. (Oxford University Press) New York, 1994; 25.
7. Weisman, Abner I. Spermatozoa and sterility, Paul B. Hoeber Inc. Medical book department of Harper Brothers, New York, 1941; 1-2.

CHAPTER
3

Sperm Morphology Classification Systems

CONTENTS

- **Earlier systems of sperm morphology classification:**
  - Williams et al. 1937
  - Hotchkiss et al. 1938
  - Macleod and Gold 1952; MacLeod 1964
- **Subsequent systems of sperm morphology classification:**
  - Eliasson 1971; 1981
  - David 1975
  - Düsseldorf 1985; 1987
- **Current systems of sperm morphology classification:**
  - WHO 1999
  - Tygerberg 1990

SYSTEMS OF CLASSIFICATION OF SPERM MORPHOLOGY

Several investigators, during the last seventy-five years, had endeavored to classify human spermatozoa on the basis of their morphological characteristics. These classification systems of sperm morphology, for the sake of convenience, can be grouped into the following three categories in order to understand their sequential development. (1) Earlier systems of sperm morphology classification. (2) Subsequent developments in the sperm morphology classification. (3) Current systems of sperm morphology classification.

EARLIER SYSTEMS OF SPERM MORPHOLOGY CLASSIFICATION

Moench and Holt (1931) had expressed an opinion that the head of spermatozoa was the biggest single source of information of the fertility status and the percentage of head abnormalities was a good indicator of the reproductive capacity of the individual. His opinion was to reign supreme for the next twenty-five years.

Williams et al., (1934) not only described the acrosome for the first time, but also divided spermatozoa into four parts, namely, head, neck, midpiece and tail regions.

The earlier systems of sperm morphology classification introduced by Williams et al., (1937), Hotchkiss et al., (1938) and MacLeod and Gold (1952, 1964) were thus entirely based on the abnormalities of sperm head.

The comparison of the earlier systems of sperm morphology classifications reveals some interesting features.

The salient features of classification of Williams et al., (1937) were the inclusion 'Pyriform' heads and 'acrosomal abnormalities' listed under sperm head defects.

On the other hand the inclusion of 'Pinheads and Round heads' under the sperm head defects was the characteristics feature of classification of Hotchkiss et al., (1938).

The unique feature of classification of MacLeod and Gold (1952) was the inclusion of 'Tapering sperms' listed under the sperm head defects. MacLeod later on (1964) modified his earlier classification by including precursor cells under the category of head defects.

The comparative features of earlier systems of sperm morphology classification are listed in Table 3.1.

Table 3.1: Summarizes the earlier systems of sperm morphology classification

EARLIER SYSTEMS OF SPERM MORPHOLOGY CLASSIFICATION

Williams et al., (1937)	*Hotchkiss et al., (1938)*	*MacLeod and Gold (1952) (1964)*
1. Normal	1. Normal	1. Normal
2. Megalosperm	2. Giant head	2. Megalosperm
3. Microsperm	————	3. Small
————	3. Pin heads	————
————	4. Round heads	————
	5. Duplicate cells	4. Duplications
————	————	5. Tapering
4. Pyriform	————	————
5. Miscellaneous: Defective head body or tail	6. Miscellaneous	6. Amorphous
6. Acrosomal abnormalities	————	————
————	————	7. Precursor cells

SUBSEQUENT SYSTEMS OF SPERM MORPHOLOGY CLASSIFICATION

Eliasson, David, and Düsseldorf made important contributions to the sperm morphology classification during the period 1971 – 1987. It must be acknowledged that these authors suggested important changes of far reaching significance in the earlier systems of classification.

CONTRIBUTION MADE BY ELIASSON

- Eliasson (1971) amended the basic classification of MacLeod (1952, 1964) by incorporating neck, midpiece and tail defects and included the additional category of "cytoplasmic droplets".
- He also emphasized the basic principle of utmost importance that the 'whole' of the spermatozoon should be assessed and a 'normal' spermatozoon should have a normal head, midpiece and tail as substantiated by actual micrometric measurements.
- He considered all 'borderline' forms as 'normal'.
- Most importantly Eliasson (1981) pointed out that an abnormal sperm may have several combined defects of head, midpiece and tail and cognizance should be taken of all such defects instead of counting one single defect.

CONTRIBUTION MADE BY DAVID

- David (1975) separated spermatozoa into two basic categories of 'Normal' and 'Abnormal' forms. The abnormal sperms were subdivided according to 'head', 'midpiece' and 'tail' abnormalities.
- This system allows a single entry of normal forms and up to four simultaneous entries for individual abnormal forms.
- This principle was later incorporated in the calculation of teratozoospermia index (TZI) recommended by WHO (1999).

CONTRIBUTION OF DÜSSELDORF

Düsseldorf (1985, 1987) introduced a new classification system of sperm morphology (Hofman & Haider 1985, Hofman et al., 1985, Hofman 1987). This clinically oriented system particularly laid emphasis on three sperm defects: (A) elongated sperm heads, (B) acrosomal defects, and (C) tail defects.

Elongated Sperm Heads

Düsseldorf further subclassified the defects of 'Elongated' sperm heads in three categories as Type HI°, Type HII° and Type HIII°, depending on the degrees and severities of elongation.
- *Type HI° defect:* Slightly elongated sperm heads with even distribution between acrosomal and post-acrosomal areas.
- *Type HII° defect:* Sperm heads with a cone shaped elongation of the post-acrosomal regions.
- *Type HIII° defect:* Sperm heads with extensive elongation of the post-acrosomal regions ending in button-like deformations.

The Acrosomal Defects

The acrosomal defects were further subdivided into two types as Type AI° and Type AII° defects.
- *Type AI° defect:* 'Small' or 'Narrowed' sperm heads with either 'small' or 'absent' acrosomes.
- *Type AII° defect:* Either small or absent acrosomes in round sperm heads with condensation of nuclear chromatin.

Defects of Sperm Tails

Three types of tail defects, designated as 1) Type I° defects, 2) Type II° defects and 3) Type III°, were included in his classification.
- *Type I° defect:* Broken tails.
- *Type II° defects:* Broken tails at the neck or midpiece region with coiling of tails.
- *Type III° defect:* Short rudimentary tails.

The salient features of subsequent systems of sperm morphology classification are tabulated in Table 3.2.

Table 3.2: Summarizes the subsequent systems of sperm morphology classification

SUBSEQUENT SYSTEMS OF SPERM MORPHOLOGY CLASSIFICATION

	Eliasson (1971, 1981)	*David (1975)*	*Düsseldorf (1985, 1987)*
1. Head defects:	1. Normal	1. Normal	1. Normal
	2. Small heads	2. Small heads	2. Too small
	3. Large head	3. Large heads	3. Too large
	4. Duplications	4. Double	4. Duplicate forms
	5. Tapered	5. Tapered	————
	6. Amorphous	6. Amorphous	————
	————	7. Thin	————
	————	8. Lysis	————
	————	————	5. Hyperelongations. TypeHI°, HII° & HIII°
	————	————	6. Acrosomal defects: AI°&AII°
2. Neck defects:	7. Neck defects	————	
3. Midpiece defects:	8. Midpiece defects	9. Cytoplasmic droplets	7. Midpiece & Tail defects
4. Tail abnormalities:	9. Tail defects	10. Bent tails	
		11. Absent tails	
		12. Short tails	
		13. Coiled tails	
		14. Double tails	8. Type I°
			9. Type II°
			10. Type III°
5. Combination of head and tail defects:	————	————	11. Combination of head and tail defects
6. Cytoplasmic droplets:	10. Cytoplasmic droplets	————	————

The Table 3.3 represents the two systems of sperm morphology classification currently in vogue.

Table 3.3: Summarizes the current systems of sperm morphology classification.

CURRENT SYSTEMS OF MORPHOLOGICAL CASSIFICATION OF HUMAN SPERMATOZOA

	WHO Classification (1999)	*Tygerberg Classification (1990)*
1. Normal Sperm (1A)	Whole sperm considered.	Whole sperm considered.
2A. Head Defects:	1. Large heads	1. Large heads
	2. Small heads	2. Small heads
	3. Tapered heads	3. Tapered / Elongated heads
	4. Pyriform heads	————
	5. Round heads	————
	6. Amorphous heads	4. Amorphous heads
	7. Vacuolated heads (More than 20% of the head area is occupied by vacuoles)	————
	8. Small acrosomes. (Acrosomes occupying less than 40% of head area.)	————
	9. Double heads	5. Duplicate heads
	Any combination of these.	6. Normal sperm heads with neck/ midpiece/or tail defects and/or cytoplasmic droplets
3. Neck Defects:	10. Bent neck and tail forms an angle greater than 90°to the long axis of the head	7. Thick necks

Contd...

Contd...

		WHO Classification (1999)	Tygerberg Classification (1990)
4.	**Midpiece Defects:**	11. Asymmetrical insertion of midpiece into the head	————
		12. Thick or irregular midpiece	8. Thickened midpiece
		13. Abnormally thin midpiece: (No mitochondrial sheath)	
		Any combination of these	9. Abnormally thin midpiece (No mitochondrial sheath)
5.	**Tail Defects:**	14. Bent tails; Bent tails forming an angle greater than 90° over any part of the tail.	10. Bent tails forming an angle greater than 90° over any part of the tail
		15. Short tails	11. Short tails
		16. Coiled tails	12. Coiled tails
		17. Irregular tails	13. Irregular tails
		18. Multiple tails	14. Loose heads (Only tails)
		19. Tails with irregular width	————
		Any combination of these	
6.	**Pin Heads:**	Not to be counted	Not to be counted
7.	**Cytoplasmic Droplets:**	20. Greater than 1/3 rd size of the sperm head	
8.	**Precursor Cells:**	Considerd abnormal	15. Precursors and 16 Unknown cells

CURRENT SYSTEMS OF SPERM MORPHOLOGY CLASSIFICATION

WHO classification (1999) and Tygerberg classification (1990) are the two methods currently in vogue for sperm morphology classification.

As WHO (1999) has adopted the 'Strict" criteria (Menkveld et al., 1990) for determining the morphological features of 'Normal spermatozoon', the difference in these two classification systems is limited to the redistribution of 'Abnormal forms' in different individual categories.

The common feature of both these systems can be described as follows. The spermatozoa are first divided into two groups: 'Normal' (whole sperm) and 'Abnormal forms'. The latter are further classified according to the abnormalities of sperm head, neck, midpiece and tail. In addition Tygerberg classification takes cognizance of "Precursor cells" and "Cells of unknown origin".

WHO CLASSIFICATION (1999)

A closer scrutiny of WHO classification (1999), which is the culmination of successive revisions of its 1980, 1987 and 1992 versions, reveals that it is a comprehensive scheme evolved after incorporating important features of earlier classification systems of MacLeod (1952,1964), Hotchkiss (1938) and David (1975).

Head Defects

The list of 'Head defects' includes important additions to the original classification of MacLeod (1952,1964). 'Pyriform heads' and 'Acrosomal defects' are included from the classification of Williams (1937) and the entity of 'Round heads' from classification of Hotchkiss (1938) is to be found listed under 'Head defects'.

Tail Defects

The entity of 'Tail defects' seems to be a modification of classification of David (1975) with additional inclusions of 'Broken tails', 'Hairpin tails' and 'Tails with irregular width'.

Important Omissions

'Loose heads' and 'Pin heads 'do not figure in WHO classification. (1999) Other cellular elements: Like 'Precursor cells', 'Macrophage cells', 'Pus cells' and 'Cells of unknown origin' are conspicuous by their absence.

Desirable Modifications

1. Under the category of (Head defects) the 8th subgroup of 'small acrosomes' ought to have been labelled as 'acrosomal defects' to make it all-inclusive to accommodate other acrosomal abnormalities.
2. There is a necessity of inclusion of a separate category for "Loose heads". The exclusion of 'Pin heads' is understandable, as these forms do not represent morphologically complete spermatozoa. But so is not the case with 'Loose sperm heads', which are simply sperms without tails. This entity of 'Loose sperm heads' should have been incorporated at least in the category of "Tail defects".
3. Likewise under the category of "Head defects" a welcome addition would have been the 10th subgroup entitled as "Spermatozoa with normal sperm heads but having defects in the region of neck, midpiece, or tail and presence of cytoplasmic droplets" In absence of a separate subgroup, such forms neither can be included in the category of 'Normal forms' (which by definition must be wholly normal) nor these sperm heads can be included in the 'Amorphous' category. This makes the calculation of "Teratozoospermia Index" difficult if not cock-eyed.

TYGERBERG CLASSIFICATION (1990)

It must be clearly understood that the word 'Strict' used in the Tygerberg's classification does not refer to the actual measurements. It only means stricter application of standards for determining 'normal' forms and distinguishing them from 'slightly abnormal' and 'borderline forms' that are to be classified as 'abnormal'.

The 'Strict' Tygerberg criteria were originally developed in 'in vivo' situations. (Van Zyl et al., 1976, 1990) and thereafter-applied in 'in vitro' situations (Kruger et al., 1986).

Tygerberg classification (Menkweld et al. 1990) is based on the modifications of classifications of MacLeod (1952), Eliasson (1971) and Freund (1966). In this classification, sperm heads are classified into seven groups as follows:

1. Normal sperms
2. Large heads
3. Small heads
4. Elongated/tapering heads
5. Duplicate heads
6. Amorphous heads
7. Normal sperm heads with neck/midpiece/and/or tail defects and/or presence of cytoplasmic droplets
   The following additional entities are also included
8. Precursors
9. Tail abnormalities
10. Neck/Midpiece abnormalities
11. Cytoplasmic droplets
12. Loose sperm heads.

Important Shortcomings of Tygerberg Classification

1. Under the "sperm head defects" there is no separate category of "acrosomal defects". Hence spermatozoa with defective and absent acrosomes (including globozoospermia) are to be included in the category of 'amorphous sperm heads'. What is more important is the exclusion of 'acrosomal defects' even in the secondary classification. This is despite the claim of Jeulin et al., (1986) that the acrosomal status is the most important criteria for the predictive value in in vitro fertilization.

2. The "pyriform sperm heads" are similarly not listed as an independent entity but are clubbed together with 'elongated/tapering heads' which is not a welcome feature. The 'elongated' sperm heads are classified in three groups (Eliasson 1971). Group 1 includes sperm heads that measure >5 μm in length with a width of 3 μm. Note that the sperm heads that are longer than the upper limits for normality and thinner than the upper limits of normal width are included in this group. Group 2 includes the sperm heads that are < 5 μm in length with a width < 2 μm. These types of sperm heads are less common. Note that the sperm heads that are shorter in length than the lower limits of normality and thinner than the lower limits for normal width are included in this group. Group 3 includes pear shaped or pyriform sperm heads. The important feature of 'pyriform' heads is sharp pointed elongation of the post acrosomal base region. Such sperm heads, though their width may often exceed 3 μm are not to be classified as "too large" as the shape of the sperm heads takes precedence over their size in the classification.

In WHO classification (1999) the total sperm abnormalities are subdivided under twenty-one different categories.

The author prefers WHO (1999) classification of sperm morphology *with inclusion and modifications suggested above*.

REFERENCE VALUES FOR NORMAL SEMEN (WHO) 1999

Volume	2 ml or more
pH	7.2 or more
Sperm concentration	20×10^6 spermatozoa /ml or more
Motility	50% or more (Rapid progressive motility and Sluggish progressive motility)
Viability	75% or more at ½ hour
Morphology	* Multicentric trials are in progress
	Data from assisted reproductive techniques suggests that as the percentage of normal sperms falls below 15% the rate of fertilization in vitro decreases.

BIBLIOGRAPHY

1. David G, Bisson JP, Cryglik F, Jaunet P, Genigon C. Anomalies morphologiques du spermatozoide humain. 1. Propositions pour un systeme de classification. J Gynecol Obstet Biol Reprod 1975; 4 (suppl. 1), 17.
2. Eliasson R. Standards for investigation for human semen. Andrologie 1971; 3: 49.
3. Eliasson R. Analysis of semen. In Burger H, DeKrester D, (eds): The Testis. New York: Raven Press, 1981;381.
4. Freund M. Standards for rating of human sperm morphology, A cooperative study. Int J Fertil 1966;11:97.
5. Hofman N, Haider SG. Naue Ergebnisse morphologischer Diagnostik der Spermatogenestörungen. Gynäkologe 1985; 18: 70.
6. Hofman N. Wege Zur Andrologie, Einführung in die Praxis. Erster Teil. (Bremerhaven: Ditzen Druck und Verlgas-GmbH, 1987.

7. Hotchkiss RS, Brunner EK, Grenely P. Semen analyses of two hundred fertile men. Amer Jour Med Sci 1938; 196: 362.

8. Jeulin C, Fenux D, Serres C, Jauannet P, Gulliet-Roso F, Belaisch-Allart, Frydman R, Testart J. Sperm factors related to failure of human in-vitro fertilization. J Reprod Fertili 1986; 76:735.

9. Kruger TF, Menkveld R, Stander FSH, Lombard CJ, Van der Merwe JP, Van Zyl JA, Smith K. Sperm morphological features as a prognostic factor in in vitro fertilizationn. Fertil Steril 1986; 46: 1118.

10. MacLeod J. Human seminal cytology as a sensitive index of germinal epithelium. Int J Fertil 1964; 9: 281.

11. Macleod J, Gold RZ. The male factor in fertility and infertility, IV Sperm morphology in fertile and infertile marriage. Fertil Steril 1952; 2: 394.

12. Menkveld R, Stander FSH, Kotz TJ. vW, Kruger TF, Van Zyl J A. The evaluation of morphological characteristics of human spermatozoa according to stricter criteria. Human Reprod 1990; 5:586.

13. Moench GL, Holt H. Sperm morphology in relation to fertility. Amer J Obstect Gynecol 1931; 22:199.

14. Van Zyl JA, Menkveld R, Kotze TJ vW, van NickeL WA. The importance of spermiograms that meet the requirements of International standard and the most important factors that influence semen parameters. Proceedings of the 17th Congress of the International Society, 1976; 2: 269. (Paris: Diffusion Dion Editerus).

15. Van Zyl JA, Kotze TJ vW, Menkveld R. Predictive value of spermatozoa morphology in natural fertilization. In Acosta, AA, Swanson RJ, Ackerman SB, Kruger TF, Van Zyl JA, Menkveld R (eds): Human Spermatozoa in Assisted Reproduction. Williams and Wilkins, Baltimore 1990; 319.

16. Williams WW. Spermatic abnormalities. New Eng J Med 1937; 217: 946.

17. Williams WW, Mac Guigan A, Carpenter HD. The staining and morphology of human spermatozoa. J Urol 1934; 32: 201.

18. World Health Organization. WHO Laboratory manual for the examination of human semen and sperm-cervical mucus interaction. 4th edn. (Cambridge: Cambridge University Press) 1999.

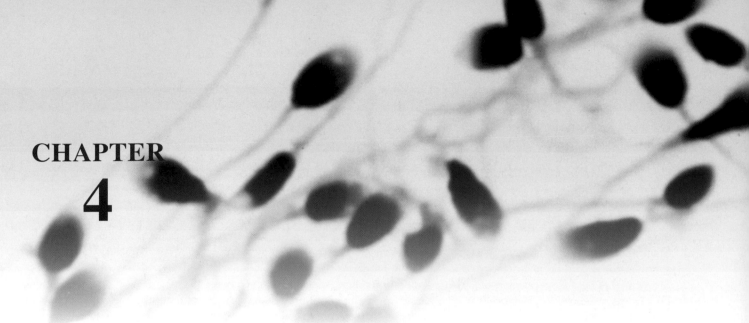

Calculation of Indices and Recording of Sperm Morphology

> ### Calculation of Indices:
>
> - Multiple Anomalies Index (MAI)
> - Teratozoospermia Index (TZI)
> - Sperm Deformity Index (SDI)
> - Procedure of Recording of Sperm Morphology
> - Calculation of Indices

CALCULATION OF INDICES

In the previous chapter a brief review of the evolution of the systems of sperm morphology classification was taken. The current systems of sperm morphology classification with their respective important features and shortcomings were also assessed.

At present there is a heavy bias in favor of 'normal spermatozoa' in the current systems of sperm morphology classification. 'Strict' Tygerberg criteria refer to the identification of 'normal forms' and their relationship with infertility, both in vivo and in vitro, situations. On the other hand WHO classification (1999) refrains from stating the permissible limits of abnormal sperms in semen samples of fertile men pending the results of multi-centric trials that are in progress. If abnormal sperms were not to figure in their relationship with infertility, then the topic of abnormal sperm morphology becomes redundant. The evaluation of the Multiple Anomalies Index (MAI) or Teratozoospermia index (TZI) and Sperm Deformity Index (SDI) assumes importance in this scenario.

1. Multiple Anomalies Index (MAI) and Teratozoospermia Index (TZI):
2. Sperm Deformity Index (SDI)

In 1971, Eliasson pointed out that abnormal spermatozoa could have multiple combined defects of head, midpiece and tail. He insisted that each of these defects must be counted separately. Jaunnet et al., (1988) used the term 'Multiple Anomalies Index '(MAI) and Mortimer (1985) referred to the same as 'Teratozoospermia Index' (TZI).

The Basic Idea of Indices

The basic aim in calculating 'MAI' or 'TZI' is to express in the form of an Index the total number of sperm abnormalities in a given number of abnormal spermatozoa. The Sperm Deformity Index (S.D.I.), on the other hand, expresses the total number of sperm abnormalities in the *total* number of spermatozoa.

Relationship with Infertility

Jaunnet et al., (1988) demonstrated that with MAI of 1.56 pregnancies in vivo did not occur but with MAI of 1.5 pregnancies did occur.

Aziz et al., (1996) found that SDI of 1.6 is the threshold for failure of fertilization.

Recording and Reporting of Sperm Morphology

Recording of sperm morphology involves double scoring, one for the primary classification the second for the secondary classification. This can be done by using two white blood cell counters, one having 10 keys and second having 8 keys. The method described below is for WHO (1999) classification as modified by the author.

The following abbreviations are used:

For primary classification of sperm head abnormalities:
1. **NS:** Normal sperm (Whole sperm)
2. **NH:** Sperms with normal heads but having defects either in the neck, midpiece region, tail region and/or with attached cytoplasmic droplets
3. **LH:** Large sperm heads
4. **SH:** Small sperm heads
5. **TP:** Tapered sperm heads
6. **PY:** Pyriform sperm heads
7. **RH:** Round sperm heads
8. **AH:** Amorphous sperm heads
9. **VH:** Vacuolated heads
10. **DH:** Sperms with two or more heads

The keys of the cell counter for the primary classification should be labelled with abbreviated forms stated above.

For the secondary classification of abnormal forms:

1. **AD:** Sperm acrosome defects
2. **ND:** Sperm neck defects
3. **MD:** Sperm midpiece defects
4. **TD:** Sperm tail defects
5. **CR:** Cytoplasmic remnants (droplets) remaining attached to the sperm
6. **OH:** Only loose sperm heads

The keys of the cell counter for the secondary classification of sperm abnormalities should be labelled with abbreviated forms stated above.

While recording, every sperm head defect is first entered in the primary classification that deals with the sperm head abnormalities. The acrosomal, neck. midpiece and tail abnormalities should be entered into the secondary classification. For example, a sperm with a tapered head, has also a small acrosome, a thick neck and two tails. Press the Key **TP** in the primary classification. Simultaneously make three entries in the secondary classification by pressing successively the Keys marked as **AD, ND and TD**. Continue recording the sperm abnormalities till the entry tally in the primary classification reaches 100. The W.B.C. cell counters are conventionally calibrated for 100 entries. When two hundred sperms are to be counted, the entries made for the first 100 sperm abnormalities should be noted down and continue the procedure to record the sperm abnormalities in the second group of 100 spermatozoa. The mean of the readings of both the entries should be taken to arrive at the percentage of sperm abnormalities.

The sperm abnormalities can also be classified by a manual method. Page 30 illustrates the format for the same. The sperm abnormalities in the semen sample of a fertile man are taken as an example. It also shows the methods for calculating the indices and briefly reports the results. In this method abbreviated names are entered in a block of 100 squares designated to the primary classification meant for recording the sperm head defects.

In the secondary classification of sperm abnormalities a tick mark (*) is entered in the requisite rows against the particular sperm abnormality.

The method is tedious and time consuming and is not suitable when large numbers of semen samples are to be examined. At best, it can be used as a stand by method if the blood cell counters are not available or not working.

Reporting the Sperm Abnormalities

The data presented in the page (page 30) should be reported as follows:

Total number of spermatozoa counted	:	100
A: Normal spermatozoa	:	23%
B: The number of abnormal spermatozoa	:	77%
1 : Spermatozoa with normal heads	:	3%
2 : Large heads	:	5%
3 : Small heads	:	16%
4 : Tapered heads	:	4%
5 : Round heads	:	5%
6 : Amorphous heads	:	33%

7	: Vacuolated heads	:	4%
8	: Double heads	:	7%
9	: Acrosomal defects	:	10%
10	: Neck defects	:	2%
11	: Midpiece defects	:	4%
12	: Tail defects	:	8%
13	: Cytoplasmic droplets	:	3%
14	: Loose heads	:	1%

CALCULATION OF MAI OR TZI

A: Total number of abnormal sperms: 77

B: Total number of sperm abnormalities:
77 in the primary classification+28 in
the secondary classification: 105
MAI or TZI: 105÷77=   1.36

Calculation of SDI

A: Total number of spermatozoa examined: 100

B: Total number of sperm abnormalities: 105
SDI = 105÷100 =   1.05

Important Note

WHO classification (1999) advises to examine at least 200 spermatozoa for the assessment of sperm morphology. However, in patients with severe oligozoospermia with sperm counts between 5 to 10 millions of spermatozoa per cu. cm, thin smears of semen may present a difficulty in counting 200 spermatozoa because of the paucity of sperm population. In such a case even the examination of less than 100 spermatozoa would suffice for the calculation of Indices as they are expressed as percentages.

DRAWBACK OF THE PRESENT RECORDING SYSTEM OF SPERM MORPHOLOGY

The method of recording of the sperm abnormalities described above suffers from a singular drawback, namely that the identity of the individual abnormalities of neck, midpiece and tail is lost as these are clubbed together simply under the neck, midpiece and tail defects. For example, the midpiece defects like bent midpiece, thick midpiece, and thin midpiece are simply recorded under the category of "midpiece defects".

To circumvent this drawback one may adopt the multiple entry system described by David et al., (1975). In this system the primary classification of head abnormalities remains unchanged. But while recording the neck, midpiece and tail defects, an individual defect is recorded separately. However, this is a manual method and the use of cell counters becomes impracticable.

Format for recording the sperm morphology: Manual method

Primary classification: Sperm head defects WHO (1999) As Modified by the author.

Abbreviations		Illustrative example (Example of 100 Sperms counted)										Total
NS	Normal Sperms	NS	LH	NS	RH	AH	AH	NS	NS	SH	AH	23%
NH	Normal Head	AH	AH	NS	NS	AH	RH	AH	VH	DH	AH	3%
LH	Large Heads	AH	NS	TP	AH	DH	NH	TP	AH	AH	NS	5%
SH	Small Heads	NH	AH	NS	SH	NH	AH	SH	AH	AH	SH	16%
TP	Tapered Heads	AH	NS	NS	DH	SH	AH	AH	SH	AH	AH	4%
RH	Round Heads	RH	VH	AH	AH	VH	SH	AH	AH	DH	SH	5%
AH	Amorphous Heads	NS	SH	NS	SH	AH	RH	NS	RH	NS	LH	33%
VH	Vacuolated Heads	NS	NS	DH	NS	TP	SH	NS	AH	AH	SH	4%
DH	Double Heads	NS	AH	SH	NS	TP	NS	AH	SH	NS	LH	7%
		AH	SH	LH	DH	AH	DH	AH	VH	SH	LH	
Total												**100**

Secondary Classification

Abbreviations			Total
AD	Acrosomal Defects **********		10
ND	Neck Defects **		2
MD	Midpiece defects ****		4
TD	Tail defects ********		8
CR	Cytoplasmic remnants (Droplets) ***		3
LH	Loose heads *		1
	Total		28

Reporting of Sperm Morphology

Normal Sperms: 23	23
Total of Abnormal Forms: (Primary classification) 100-23 =	77
Total Sperm Abnormalities: 77+28	105
M.A.I.= Total Sperm Abnormalities ÷Total number of Abnormal sperms counted. 105÷77	**1.36**

BIBLIOGRAPHY

1. Aziz N, Buchan L, Taylor C, Kingland CR, Lewis-Jones I. The sperm deformity index: a reliable predictor of the outcome of oocyte fertilization in vitro. Fertil Steril 1996; 66: 95.
2. David G, Bisson JP, Czyglik F, Jaunnet P, Hrenigon C. Anomolies morphologiques du spermatozoíde humain, (1) Propsitions pour un systëme de classification. J. Gynecol. Obstet Biol Reprod 1975; 4 Suppl. 1: 17.
3. Eliason R. Standards for investigation for human semen. Andrologie 1971; 3: 49.
4. Jauannet P, Ducot B, Feneux D, Spira A. Male factor and the likelihood of pregnancy in infertile couples.1, Study of sperm characteristics. Int. J Androl 1988; 11: 379.
5. Mortimer D. The male factor in infertility. Part I. Semen analysis. In: Current problems in Obstetrics, Gynecology and Fertility (ed): JM Leventhal, Chicago, Illinois Year book Medical Publishers, Inc. 1985; 1.
6. World Health Organization. WHO Laboratory manual for the examination of human semen and sperm-cervical mucus interaction. 4th edn. (Cambridge: Cambridge University Press), 1999.

CHAPTER 5

Staining Methods for Sperm Morphology

The quest for an ideal staining method for sperm morphology continues

Requirements:

- Fixation should produce minimal distortion and shrinkage of the cellular elements.
- Ability to stain viscous semen samples.
- Simple procedure suitable for even small laboratories.
- Method should be least time consuming, cost effective, reproducible and with easy availability of stains.
- In the stained smears the background should be free from granular debris.
- The spermatozoa and the other cellular elements like precursor cells of spermatozoa, macrophage cells, pus cells, epithelial cells, parasites like trichomonas and bacteria should be nicely stained obviating the need to use of any other additional supplementary stain.
- Different parts of spermatozoon like the head (including the acrosome and post acrosomal parts of the sperm nucleus), neck, midpiece and tail should be distinctly stained.
- For the proper identification of cellular elements a differential acidophilic/basophilic stain like Papanicolaou stain is desirable.
- The stained slides should show minimal fading of colors on storage.

Such an ideal method is as yet a dream unfulfilled.

STAINING METHODS FOR SEMEN SMEARS

The different staining methods used for the assessment of sperm morphology and sperm viability are summarized in Table 5.1. For the details of the staining methods please refer Appendix-1.

Table 5.1: Staining methods for studying morphology and viability of spermatozoa	
Staining Methods	*Stains Used*
A. FOR SPERM VIABILITY	
1. Stained preparations.	a) Eosin – Nigrosin stain (Blom 1950 a) (for Bulls).
	b) Eosin – Nigrosin stain (Eliasson 1977).
2. Supravital staining.	a) Eosin Y stain (Eliasson & Streichl 1971).
	b) Eosin Y stain (WHO 1987).
3. Supravital staining of the cellular elements in semen.	Phadke (1978).
B. FOR SPERM MORPHOLOGY	
1. Routine staining methods.	a) Eosin- Nigrosin stain.
	b) Hematoxylin – Eosin stain.
	c) Rose Bengal – Toluidine blue stain.
	d) Papanicolaou stain.
	e) Shorr's stain.
2. For leukocytes in semen.	Gimsa stain.
3. Quick methods.	a) Diff Quick
	b) Spermac
4. Pre- stained slides.	Testsimplets® Testimplets®

This section gives an overview of the current staining methods for sperm morphology and highlights their scope, specificity, advantages and shortcomings.

The phase contrast microscopy, though not a staining method is included in this section to make it comprehensive. The important staining methods are illustrated in the Atlas.

FOR SPERM VIABILIY

A distinction must be made between the motility and the viability of spermatozoa. Non-moving sperms may be dead or just 'dormant'. A sperm may be viable but non-motile due to several factors such as cold shock, increased viscosity of semen, changes in the pH of the medium, collection of semen in a rubber condom or a wet container, etc.

The diagnosis of 'necrozoospermia' (all sperms dead) should only be made after confirming the status of sperm viability by Eosin-Nigrosin stain.

According to the author the second situation for the application of this method is for the assessment of the viability status of spermatozoa recovered from the cervical canal during the post coital test.

Stained Preparations

a. *Eosin – Nigrosin stain (Blom 1950 a) (For Bulls):* The Eosin – Nigrosin staining method described by Blom (1950a) for sperm viability has withstood the test of time and remains the method of choice. It is based on his classical observation namely that the aqueous solution of Eosin cannot penetrate the living spermatozoa. A background stain of Nigrosin enables the easier identification of unstained (live) spermatozoa. While interpreting the results any red or totally non-white sperms are regarded as dead sperms. The unstained 'white' sperms are regarded as living sperms.

b. *Eosin – Nigrosin stain (Eliasson 1977):* This is essentially a minor variant of Blom's method. Instead of 5% aqueous solution of Eosin B (bluish shade) used in the Blom's method, Eliasson has advocated the use of 1% aqueous solution of Eosin Y. Rest of the staining procedure is identical.

Supravital Staining Methods

a. *Eosin Y stain (Eliasson & Streichl 1971):* The supravital staining method described by Eliasson and Treichl (1971) and the method described in WHO Manual (1987, 1999) are almost similar and hence may be considered as identical despite minor variations. Instead of 0.5% solution of Eosin Y prepared in 0.9% normal saline, as in WHO methods (1987, 1999), these authors have advocated the use of 0.5% solution of Eosin Y prepared in 0.15 M phosphate buffer (pH 7.4). Otherwise the rest of staining procedure is identical. The air-dried smears are examined under a 'negative 'phase contrast microscope. The viable cells appear 'bluish' and dead cells appear 'bright yellow'.

b. *Eosin Y stain (WHO 1987):* In this method one drop of freshly liquefied semen is thoroughly mixed with one drop of 0.5% solution of Eosin Y prepared in normal saline. After couple of minutes' one drop, from Eosin Y – semen mixture, is transferred to another slide and covered with a cover slip. The cover slip preparation is examined under a high power (x 40) of either a bright field or phase contrast microscope. The dead sperms are stained red and the living sperms remain unstained.

Both of these, so called, "Supravital staining methods are in reality methods for differentiating the "Living" from "Dead" spermatozoa. It is not appropriate to call them "Supravital staining methods", for a real supravital staining method involves staining of the cells in living condition. The staining of nuclei indicates the death of the cells.

Both of these methods depend on the use of a "Negative" or "Positive" phase contrast microscope that may not be available in an average laboratory. Similarly, like Blom's stain, the cellular elements in semen other than the spermatozoa cannot be studied. Besides, the slides thus prepared cannot be stored for future reference.

Supravital Staining of Cellular Elements in Semen

Phadke (1978) has described a supravital staining method to identify the cellular elements in semen. Precursors of spermatozoa are often mistaken for pus cells by less experienced technicians. Unnecessary antibiotic therapy is administered based on these erroneous tests. In this test the cellular elements in semen are stained in living condition. Staining of the nucleus indicates the death of the cell. It permits easy identification of spermiophage cells, spermatocytes, leukocytes and trichomonas.

FOR SPERM MORPHOLOGY

Routine Staining Methods

Eosin-Nigrosin Stain

Apart from its use in the assessment of sperm viability, the Eosin-Nigrosin stain is very helpful for the assessment of sperm morphology as well. The different parts of the sperm, i.e. the head, acrosome, and neck, midpiece and tail are easily discernible. Various abnormalities of acrosomes pertaining to their size, shape and position together with the presence of lesions like cysts, vacuoles, the areas of localized condensation and the invagination of acrosome into the nucleus are observed with ease and clarity. The same is true for abnormalities of sperm neck, midpiece and tail.

In fact, Glezerman and Bartoov (1993) prefer to rely exclusively on this stain for assessing the sperm morphology.

This simple and inexpensive method, within the reach of a smallest laboratory, remains the only reliable method for the simultaneous assessment of sperm viability and morphology. Moreover the stained slides can be mounted with DPX and preserved for future reference.

However, this method has a singular drawback. It is not suitable for the study of the cellular elements in semen. Unfortunately the WHO Manual (1999) has not emphasized the usefulness of this method for assessing the sperm morphology.

In the Eosin-Nigrosin stained preparations, the background is dark. In order to circumvent this disadvantage, the author prefers to use 5% aqueous solution of Eosin Y ((In place of 1% aqueous solution of Eosin B) and 1% aqueous solution of Nigrosin (In place of 10% aqueous solution of Nigrosin) described in the original staining method without jeopardizing the efficacy of the stain.

Hematoxylin and Eosin Stain

H and E stain is readily available in all pathology laboratories. It serves as a good stain for sperm morphology. In the H and E stained seminal smears the post acrosomal portions of the sperm nuclei, are stained blue. The cytoplasm of cells, acrosomes and the tails of spermatozoa are stained pink. Likewise the free residual bodies and the remnants of cytoplasm remaining attached to the various parts of spermatozoa are also stained pink. Moreover, the viscous semen samples can also be stained.

Unfortunately, there is a likelihood of diffusion of the nuclear stain in the cell cytoplasm resulting in indistinct demarcation between the two. The acrosomal lesions are not seen with ease and clarity. The identification of the cellular elements other than spermatozoa is solely dependant on their nuclear characteristics alone. Hence Papanicolaou or Shorr's stain is preferred in the sperm morphology assessment for easier identification of the other cellular elements.

Rose Bengal and Toluidine Blue Stain

This staining method, invented by the author, is being introduced for the first time in this Atlas. It differs radically from the other conventional staining methods wherein the semen smears are stained first with a nuclear stain and after differentiation a counter stain is applied to stain the cytoplasm. It is based on the author's original observation, namely that the Toluidine blue O stain replaces the nuclear stain of Rose Bengal from the cells in the semen smears previously stained with a specially prepared Rose Bengal stain. As a result of this, the cytoplasm of cells is stained pink while their nuclei are stained deep blue or purple. There is no diffusion of the nuclear stain in cell cytoplasm thereby resulting in excellent demarcation between the two. The acrosomes and tails of spermatozoa retain the pink color while the post acrsomal portions of sperm nuclei are stained deep purple or blue. Various acrosomal lesions like vacuoles, cysts, areas of localized condensation and acrosomal invagination into the nucleus etc. are easily perceived. Likewise nuclear defects like vacuoles, acrosomal or cytoplasmic invaginations into the nucleus are easily identified. The cytoplasmic remnants remaining attached to the different parts of spermatozoa and the free residual bodies are stained pink. It is an excellent stain for the leukocytes and macrophage cells present in semen. Besides, the cytoplasmic organelle and bacteria together with parasites present in the semen are stained with Toluidine blue.

Although like in the H and E stain the identification of cellular elements is solely based on their nuclear characteristics alone, it is seldom necessary to use Papanivolaou or Shorr stain for this purpose. This simple staining method is eminently suitable for an average pathology laboratory with a lesser workload of semen tests.

Papanicolaou Stain

Papanicolaou (1942) originally published a new staining procedure for staining the vaginal smears. With suitable modifications, in fact as many as the number of investigators, this stain is adapted for sperm morphology. Papanicolaou stain is essentially an acidophilic/basophilic stain and stains the cell cytoplasm differentially. This is extremely useful for discriminating the germinal from non-germinal cells. Because of its high alcoholic contents, the staining of the cells is delicately transparent and the details of nuclear chromatin are well revealed. The Papanicolaou stain offers more flexibility in that the duration of the counter stains can be varied.

In the seminal smears stained with this stain the sperm head is stained pale blue in the acrosomal region and dark blue in the post acrosomal region. The midpiece may show some red staining. The tails are also stained blue or reddish. The cytoplasmic droplets attached to the different parts of spermatozoa as well as the free residual bodies are stained pink. The germinal cells have pink cytoplasm while the non-germinal cells including leukocytes and macrophages have greenish blue cytoplasm. The epithelial cells are variably stained (WHO 1999).

There are certain drawbacks of this stain. The tails of spermatozoa are not stained distinctly, the acrosomal lesions are not perceived with clarity and the nuclei of the cellular elements are often masked by the counter stain and consequently appear indistinct.

Shorr's Stain

Shorr (1941) had described a new staining technique for vaginal smears. It was essentially a modification of Masson's satin. With suitable modifications it is adapted for sperm morphology.

Shorr's stain was widely used in France for many years. It is being used by increasing number of andrology laboratories and those working with IVF programs following the work of Jeulin et al., (1986)

Original Shorr's stain essentially gave two colors, bright red and greenish blue. The nuclear details were not satisfactory. De Neef - Pundel (1965) modified the original Shorr's stain to overcome its deficiencies. The modification involved the initial staining with Harris Hematoxylin. In addition the stain itself contains Aniline blue, which stains the nuclei blue. This is supplementary to the blue stained nuclei of Harris Hematoxylin.

Shorr's stain is considered to be particularly useful in evaluating abnormalities of sperm heads and acrosomes. Haidi and Schill (1993) have claimed that the tails of spermatozoa are either stained red (normal) or green (indicating that the tail is not viable). Their claim has not been substantiated. The staining characteristics of Shorr's stain are identical to that of Papanicolaou stain.

Shorr's stain has a fixed composition. Because of its simplicity it is preferable to Papanocolaou stain in sperm morphology assessment. In fact, the Papanicolaou stain and de Neef – Pundel modification of Shorr's stain are the twin methods recommended for staining cytology smears (Raphael 1976). In this Atlas De Neef – Pundel modification of Shorr's stain is used.

For Leukocytes in Semen

Gimsa Stain

Gimsa stain per se is not recommended for studying sperm morphology but is claimed to be useful in evaluating different types of white blood cells present in semen. Even in its limited application it is superseded by Papanicolaou stain. WHO Manual (1999) has rightfully refrained from mentioning it.

Quick Methods

Diff-Quick Stain

Kruger et al., (1987) introduced this stain for assessing sperm morphology. With this stain the acrosomal region of sperm head is stained pale purple, the post acrosomal portion of the sperm nucleus, midpiece and tail are stained dark purple. Apart from the prohibitive cost, in the semen smears stained with this method the size of the sperm head is larger and the background is darkly stained. Papanicolaou or Shorr stain is decidedly superior to Diff-Quick stain. Ready to use staining sets for this method are available. (Cat. No. B 4132-1, Allegiance Healthcare Corp. Mc Grow Park, Illinois, 60085-6787 USA).

Spermac Stain

Oettle (1986) had described this stain for assessing the sperm morphology. In the slides stained with Spermac stain, the acrosomal region of the sperm head, midpiece and tail are stained green and the post acrosomal portion of the sperm nucleus is stained red. The semen smears stained with Spermac stain share the same drawbacks of Diff-Quick stain.

The stain is commercially available. (Stain Enterprise, POHOX 4 Z, Koelenhorf, 7605. Republic of South Africa.)

Prestained Slides

Testsimplets®

Testsimplets ready-for-use microscope slides are prestained with N-methylene blue and cresyl violet acetate. The staining procedure is reliable, fast and makes complicated staining methods and equipment redundant.

The procedure is very simple. Apply 5 µl (0.005 ml) of freshly liquefied semen to the center of the stained portion of the slide. Place the provided cover slip and press it gently to spread uniformly the drop of semen in a thin layer. Seal the edges of the cover slip with a nail paint. Allow to remain the slide at room temperature for 30 minutes. Examine under oil immersion. The slides thus prepared are stable for 24 hours.

The acrosomes, mipieces and tails of spermatozoa are stained red and the post acrosomal portions of sperm nuclei blue. In the case of the other cellular elements the nuclei are stained blue and the cytoplasm red. Good pictures of spermatozoa as well as other cells in semen, stained with Testsimplets® are published by Adelman and Cahil (1989).

However, the testsimplets® are not suitable for viscous semen samples and the prepared slides cannot be stored.

(Prestained ready-for-use microscope slides are available from Boehringer Mannheim GMbH 6800, Mannheim 31 Germany.)

BIBLIOGRAPHY

1. Adelman MA, Cahil EM. Atlas of Sperm Morphology. ASCP Press. American Society of Clinical Pathologists. Chicago, 1989.
2. Blom E. A one minute live dead sperm stain by means of eosin – nigrosin. Fertil Steril 1950a; 1: 176.
3. De Neef JC. Clinical Endocrine Cytology. Hoeber Medical Division, Harper and Row, New York 1965.
4. Eliasson R. Supravital staining of human spermatozoa. Fertil Steril 1977; 28: 1275.
5. Eliasson R, Treichl L. Supravital staining of human spermatozoa. Fertil Steril 1971; 22: 134.
6. Glezerman, Marek and Bartoov Benjamin. Semen analysis in Infertility Male and Female (eds.) Insler, VS and Lunenfield, B Churchill Livingstone, London, 1993; 295.
7. Haidi G, Schill WB. Sperm morphology in fertile men. Arch Androl 1993; 31: 153.
8. Jeulin C, Fenux D, Serres C, Jauannet P, Gulliet-Roso F, Belaisch-Allart, Frydman R and Testart J. Sperm factors related to failure of human in-vitro fertilization. J Reprod Fertil, 1986; 76: 735.
9. Kruger TF, Acosta AA, Simmons KF, Swanson RJ, Matta JF, Veeik LL, Morshedi M, Brugo S. New method of evaluating sperm morphology with predictive value for semen. Urolog 1987; 30:(3), 248.
10. Oettle EE. Using a new acrosome stain to evaluate sperm morphology. Vet Med 1986; 8: 263.
11. Papanicolaou GN. A new procedure for staining vaginal smears. Science 1942; 95:438.
12. Phadke AM. Neutral Red staining for cellular elements in the semen. Andrologia 1978; 10: 80.
13. Raphael SS. Cytology. In Lynch's medical laboratory technology: 3rd ed. Raphael, SS (ed). WB Saunders Company, Philadelphia 1977.
14. World Health Organization. WHO Laboratory manual for the examination of human semen and sperm-cervical mucus interaction. 2nd edn. (Cambridge: Cambridge University Press) 1987.
15. World Health Organization. WHO Laboratory manual for the examination of human semen and sperm-cervical mucus interaction. 4th edn. (Cambridge: Cambridge University Press) 1999.

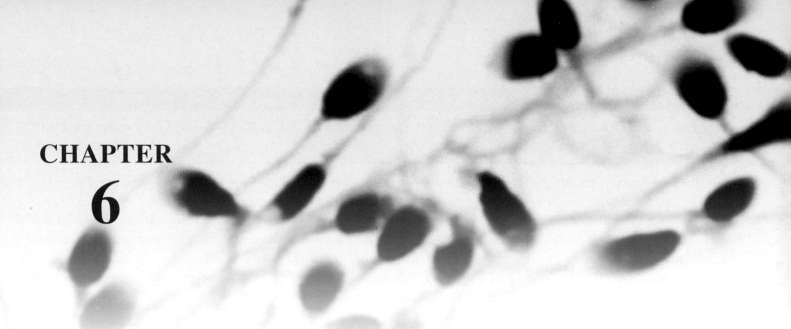

CHAPTER
6

Introduction to the Pictorial Atlas of Sperm Morphology

PICTORIAL ATLAS OF SPERM MORPHOLOGY

- Scope and limitations
- Electron microscopy pictures are not included
- Staining methods and magnification used
- Selection of the material
- Pictorial atlas for sperm morphology

One picture speaks of hundred words! So says a proverb. This is verily true regarding sperm morphology. Any detailed description of various sperm abnormalities, however, accurate and painstakingly penned, cannot replace pictures depicting various sperm abnormalities. A picture is imprinted in the memory of an individual and creates a long lasting impression. An elaborate description of various sperm abnormalities, apart from becoming boring and unintelligible, is apt to be forgotten leaving at most a faded memory about the topic read.

This 'Pictorial Atlas' is compiled not only to illustrate the different sperm abnormalities incorporated in WHO classification (1999) but also includes the sperm abnormalities described in Tygerberg classification and those found in the other classification systems, e.g. Düsseldorf, Menkveld etc, in order to present a synthetic compendium. Every effort is made to include the sperm abnormalities that are needed to be known to understand the current systems of sperm morphology classification. Additional pictures are selected to illustrate certain other lesions. This is particularly true of acrosomal abnormalities, which are either totally neglected or at best are summarily dealt with scant respect in both of the current classification systems.

The varieties of 'amorphous spermatozoa' are innumerable and it is foolhardy to illustrate them all. However, certain interesting and unique pictures are included in this 'Atlas' in order to make readers aware of limitless varieties this group embraces and to stimulate their interest.

Pictures of certain nuclear and acrosomal defects, though they remain neglected at present, find place in this collection. Likewise 'Pin headed' spermatozoa are represented because of their rarity and incurability.

It was a formidable task to select the characteristic pictures, from thousands of microphotographs in the author's collection, for inclusion in this 'Atlas' keeping in mind the riders of page and cost limits. A certain amount of repetition is unavoidable for which the author begs the reader's tolerance.

Electron Microscopy and TEM pictures are not included because of dual reasons. The author himself is not well versed with Electron Microscopy and very few, if any, of the clinicians would be. These tools offer fantastic details beyond the comprehension of average clinician who seldom would be handling these sophisticated tools. However, the information gained from these studies is incorporated in this Atlas wherever found necessary.

All the pictures depicted in this 'Atlas' are oil immersion microphotographs suitably magnified without compromising the quality and details.

The staining method selected is the author's Rose Bengal and Toluidine blue staining method. In the smears of semen stained with this method the background is free from debris, the different parts of spermatozoa are beautifully stained and the acrosomal and nuclear details are discerned with clarity. This does not imply that the other staining methods used world over are in any way inferior. For illustrating certain acrosomal and nuclear details Eosin Nigrosin stain (Blom' method) for sperm viability is selected.

Each picture has its own narration that includes the relevant selected information pooled from the available scientific data. A careful study of the pictures with their accompanying narrations will be a rewarding exercise for new entrants in this field obviating the necessity of undertaking a laborious search of scattered literature. At places the author has ventured to voice his own opinions based on his experience.

The preceding sections were intended to brief the readers regarding the anatomical structural details of spermatozoon and to give a concise account of sperm morphology and its importance, evolution with controversial points involved therein. The classification systems of sperm morphology, their salient features, evolutionary changes they had undergone and calculation of various indices were also dealt with. Equipped with this background, the reader is now in a position to study the 'Pictorial Atlas' of sperm morphology.

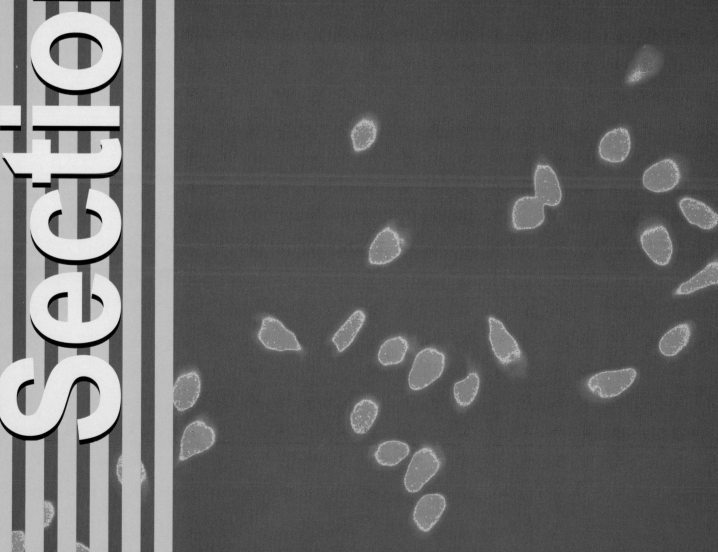

Section 2

Pictorial Atlas of
Sperm Morphology

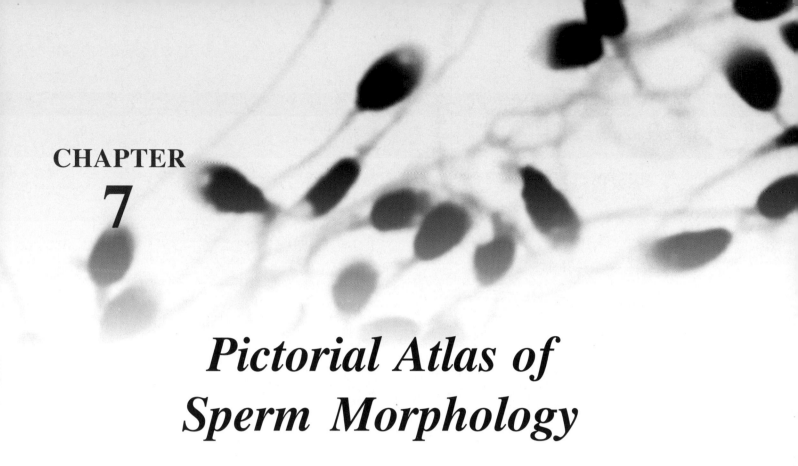

CHAPTER
7

Pictorial Atlas of Sperm Morphology

The subject of human sperm morphology is classified according to the following topics.

TOPICS

- Staining methods
- Diagrammatic representation of sperm abnormalities
- 1. Normal spermatozoa
- 1-A. sperm head defects
- 2-B. Defects of sperm acrosomes
- 3. Defects of sperm neck
- 4. Defects of sperm midpiece
- 5. Defects of sperm tail
- 6. Miscellaneous defects.

EOSIN-NIGROSIN STAIN

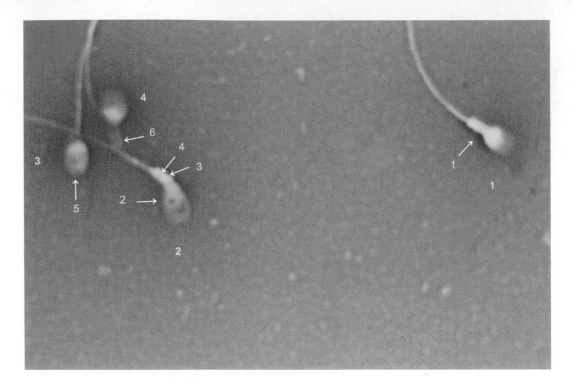

Figure 7.1: Eosin-Nigrosin stain (Oil immersion × 5000)

The Eosin-Nigrosin staining method, described by Blom (1950a), has withstood the test of time. It is based on his observation of a singular importance, namely that, the 5% aqueous solution of Eosin B has the capacity to penetrate the dead sperms which in turn are stained pink, while the living sperms remain unstained and appear white. This uncomplicated method nicely discriminates the different regions of the sperm cell.

The above picture illustrates one living and three dead sperms.

Number 1: A living sperm with a normal head has a thickened neck and midpiece (Arrow 1) but the tail is normal.

Number 2: A large sperm head shows the presence of a nuclear vacuole. (Arrow 2). The neck is thickened (Arrow 3) and the midpiece is irregular (Arrow 4).

Number 3: A normal sperm head exhibits an acrosomal vacuole (Arrow 5).

Number 4: A sperm with a normal head has a bent tail (Arrow 6).

HEMATOXYLIN AND EOSIN STAIN

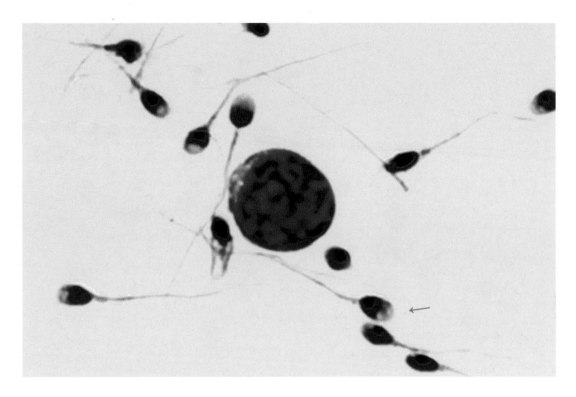

Figure 7.2: Hematoxylin and Eosin stain (Oil immersion × 5000)

In this H and E, stained smear of semen the acrocomes of spermatozoa are stained pale pink and the post acrosomal portions of the sperm nuclei are stained deep blue. The midpieces and the tails of spermatozoa are easily identifiable. The cytoplasmic droplets attached to sperms and the free residual bodies are stained pink. The acrosomal vacuoles (Arrow) are discernible.

At the center is seen a primary spermatocyte measuring 14.2 µm in diameter with its leptotene nucleus almost filling the cell.

H and E stain is routinely used in all laboratories and thus is readily available. However, the identification of the cellular elements is based entirely on the nuclear characteristics, and the size and shape of the cells.

The Papanicoloau stain has the additional advantage in that it stains the cell's cytoplasm differentially, either acidophilic or basophilic, which is of utmost importance in the identification of the cell types.

ROSE BENGAL AND TOLUIDINE BLUE STAIN

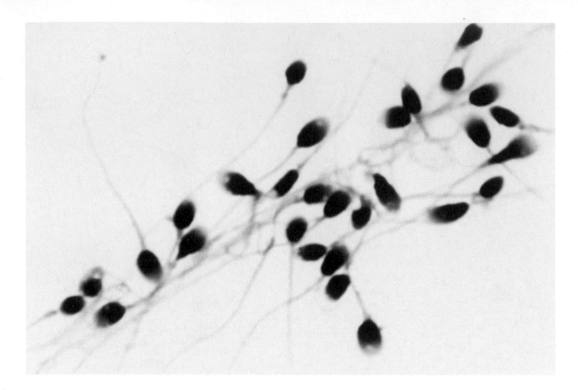

Figure 7.3: Rose Bengal and Toluidine blue stain (Oil immersion × 5000)

The smear of semen stained with author's Rose Bengal and Toluidine blue staining technique is illustrated here. With this method that is based on dye replacement, the acrosomes of spermatozoa and spermatids together with the cytoplasm of all the cells are stained pink. The post acrosomal parts of the sperm nuclei and spermatids, (-and also the nuclei of other cells), are stained deep purple or blue.

This method offers clear-cut distinction between the acrosomes and post acrosomal parts of the sperm nuclei and the junction line between the two. The vacuoles present in the acrosomes and/or in the nuclei of sperms are easily discernible.

The abnormalities of acrosomes are easily appreciated. Fine lesions like acrosomal and nuclear cysts, areas of localized condensation of acrosome and invaginations into the nucleus are easily definable. The tail abnormalities become obvious. The background is free from debris. The cellular elements can be identified by their shape, size and nuclear characteristics.

PAPANICOLAOU STAIN

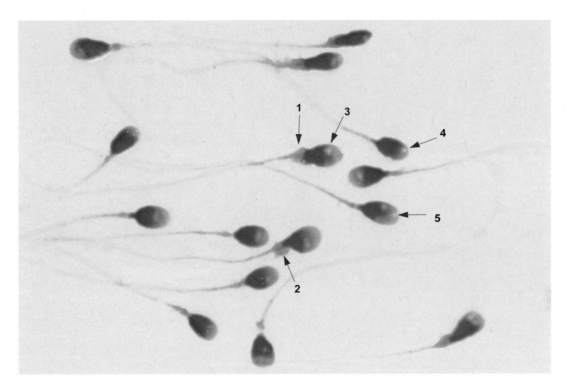

Figure 7.4: Papanicolaou stain (Oil immersion × 5000)

Papanicolaou stain is extensively used in andrology laboratories. The WHO Manual (1999) recommends this stain for sperm morphology.

With this stain the sperm head is stained pale blue in the acrosomal region and dark blue in the post-acrosomal region. The midpiece and tail are stained blue or reddish. The cytoplasmic droplets and extrusion residues, usually located behind the head and around the midpiece are stained pink (Arrows' 1 and 2). The nuclear and acrosomal vacuoles appear as pale stained areas (Arrows' 3, 4 and 5).

There are several advantages of this stain. First it is suitable for viscous semen samples. Second, being acidophilic/basophilic stain, the cell cytoplasm is differentially stained. In general, the cytoplasm of the spermatogenic cells is stained pink. The cytoplasm of macrophages, pus cells and Sertoli cells is stained bluish green. The cytoplasm of the epithelial cells is variably stained.

In better stained preparations the tails are stained pink.

SHORR'S STAIN

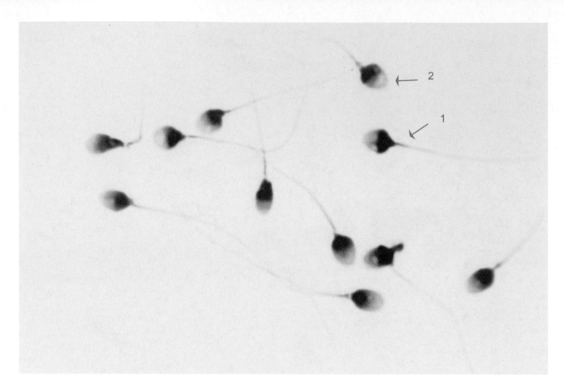

Figure 7.5: Modified Shorr's stain (Oil immersion × 5000)

This picture illustrates a semen smear stained with modified Shorr's stain. Note that the acrosomes of spermatozoa are stained pale blue and the post acrosomal portions of the sperm nuclei are stained deep blue. This is consistent with the results of the staining method described in WHO Manual and the findings of Meschede et al., (1993).

There is some red staining at the midpiece region (Arrow 1). The sperm tails are stained pale pink or blue. The acrosomal vacuoles are represented by unstained white spots (Arrow 2).

The general appearance of the seminal smear stained with Shorr's stain is similar to the one stained with Papanicolaou stain.

SUPRAVITAL STAINING OF A SPERMIOPHAGE CELL

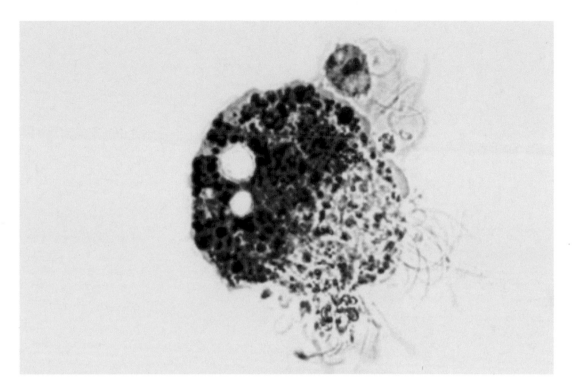

Figure 7.6: Phadke's neutral red stain (Oil immersion × 5000)

A giant binucleate spermiophage cell is stained supravitally with Neutral Red. (Phadke 1978) The cell has a diameter of 55.5 microns and the two nuclei appear as two unstained white areas at 9 and 10 o'clock position. The cell is loaded with Neutral Red granules and globules which appear bright red or blackish red. Numerous ingested sperm heads are seen in the lower part of the cell. The tails of spermatozoa are seen emerging on the right.

Supravital staining involves staining of a cell in living condition in vitro. The staining of the nucleus indicates the death of a cell.

The spermiophage cells have the unique ability of absorbing Neutral Red from weak solutions and concentrating and storing it in their cytoplasm in the form of large globules and small granules. This is an active biological process different from passive staining.

SPERMATOZOA UNDER PHASE CONTRAST MICROSCOPE

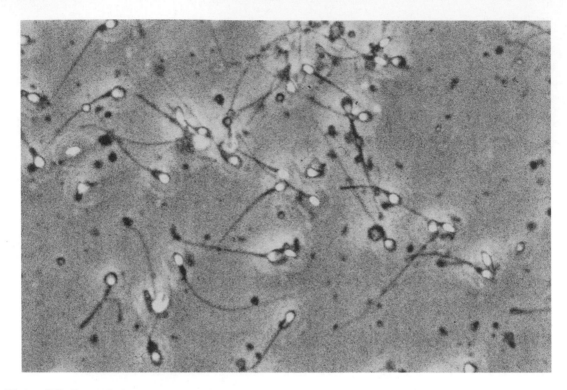

Figure 7.7: Ergaval phase contrast microscope with Planeacromat objective 40 X (Magnification × 2000)

Phase contrast microscopy is a useful tool for studying sperm morphology, especially when large number of semen samples are to be examined.

A drop of distilled water is added to a drop of semen to immobilize the sperms. The cover slip preparation is examined under 40 x-phase objective with a yellow green filter.

Gross sperm abnormalities, especially the tail defects, are easily identifiable. The sperm nuclei appear yellow, the acrosomes and the necks appear blue or purple and the tails appear purple. The other cells have blue or green nuclei and their cytoplasm appears purple.

Oil immersion objective can also be used but it becomes cumbersome to study the morphology as the sperms are floating and their tails may not be in the same focal plane.

The major disadvantage of this method is that the cover slip preparation cannot be preserved.

SPERM HEAD DEFECTS

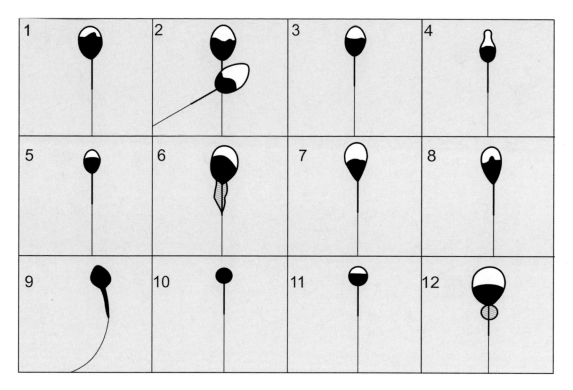

Figure 7.8: Normal and abnormal sperm heads

Numbers 1, 2 and 3: Normal sperms.
Number 4: A normal sperm in a lateral view.
Number 5: A small sperm head.
Number 6: A large sperm head with cytoplasm attached at the midpiece region.
Number 7: A pyriform sperm head.
Number 8: A tapered sperm head.
Number 9: A microsperm without acrosome and with thickened midpiece.
Number 10: A round headed sperm without acrosome (Globozoospermia)
Number 11: A round headed sperm with acrosome.
Number 12: A large round headed sperm with cytoplasm attached at the midpiece region.

DEFECTS OF SPERM HEAD

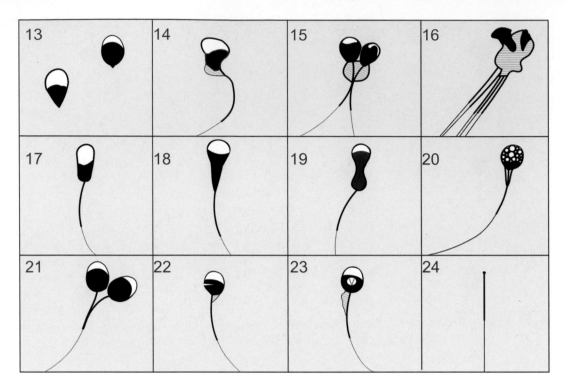

Figure 7.9: Different types of sperm head defects

Number 13: Loose sperm heads.

Number 14: Amorphous head, a thick post acrosomal portion of the nucleus, a thickened neck and a bent midpiece.

Number 15: Duplicate or conjoined form.

Number 16: Amorphous flattened head, thickened midpiece and multiple tails.

Number 17: Elongated sperm head. (Düsseldorf type HI°)

Number 18: Cone shaped elongation of the post acrosomal portion of the nucleus. (Düsseldorf type HII°)

Number 19: A Dumbbell shaped sperm head. (Düsseldorf type HIII°)

Number 20: A vacuolated sperm head.

Number 21: A double headed sperm.

Number 22: A sperm head with a cytoplasmic invagination into the nucleus.

Number 23: A sperm head with a normal nuclear vacuole.

Number 24: A pin headed sperm.

DEFECTS OF SPERM NECK, MIDPIECE AND TAIL.

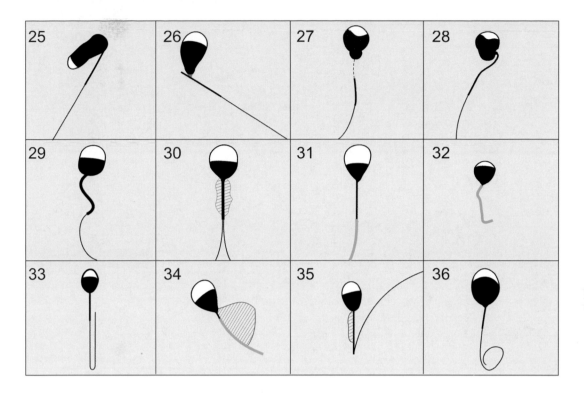

Figure 7.10: Defects of sperm neck, midpiece and tail

Number 25: An elongated head, thickened neck and a bent midpiece.

Number 26: A sperm with a pyriform head and a noninserted tail.

Number 27: A sperm with an amorphous head with a thickened neck and a thin midpiece at the beginning.

Number 28: A sperm with an amorphous head with an abnormally attached midpiece.

Number 29: A large head, with a thickened midpiece ab-axially attached.

Number 30: A sperm with a large head with attached cytoplasm at the midpiece region and two tails.

Number 31: A sperm with a large pyriform head and a thickened tail.

Number 32: A sperm with a small head and with a tadpole tail.

Number 33: A sperm with a small head with a hairpin defect of tail.

Number 34: A sperm with a pyriform head and short tail that has cytoplasmic remnants attached to it.

Number 35: A small sperm head with a bent tail.

Number 36: A sperm with a large head and a curled tail.

A NORMAL SPERM

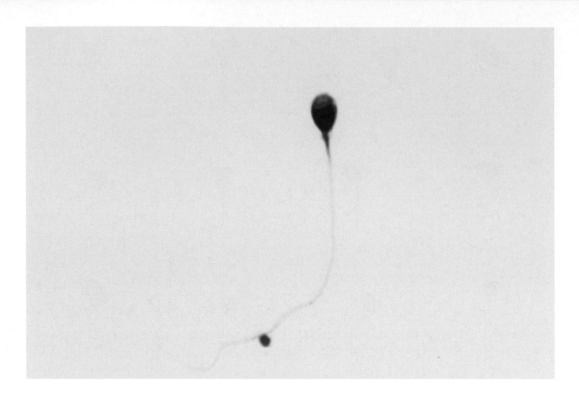

Figure 7.11: Rose Bengal and Toluidine blue stain (Oil immersion × 5000)

This picture illustrates a normal sperm. Note that the sperm head is oval in shape and is covered anteriorly by pink stained acrosome. The post-acrosomal portion of the nucleus is stained deep purple. The slight narrowing of the post-acrosomal portion of the nucleus is to be considered as normal.

The sperm head has smooth margins. It measures 4.2 μm in length and 2.8 μm in width. The length to a width ratio is 1.5. The acrosome is normal. The junction of acrosome and the nucleus is clearly seen. The midpiece measures 7.5 μm in length and is normal. The tail is centrally attached to the nucleus and is normal.

NORMAL SPERMATOZOA

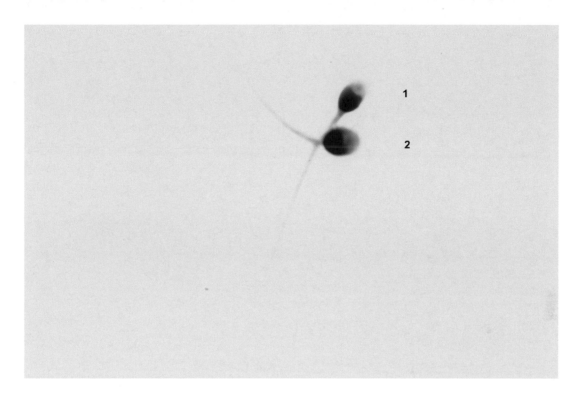

Figure 7.12: Rose Bengal and Toluidine blue stain (Oil immersion × 5000)

At first glance it would appear that a normal and large sperm head is depicted in this picture. However, the measurements taken with a micrometer confirm that both sperm heads are normal.

Number 1: This is a normal sperm head. It is oval in shape and has an acrosome covering approximately 30% of its area. The junction line between the acrosome and the post acrosomal portion of the nucleus is clear cut and distinct. The sperm head measures 4.35 µm in length and 2.90 µm in width. The ratio of length to width is 1.5 that is normal.

Number 2: This sperm head is oval in shape and has a normal acrosome covering about 30% of its area. The junction line between the acrosome and the post acrosomal portion of the nucleus is clear-cut and distinct. The head measures 4.95 µm in length and 3.15 µm in width. The length to a width ratio is 1.57 that is within normal limits.

A BORDERLINE SPERM AND A LARGE HEADED SPERM

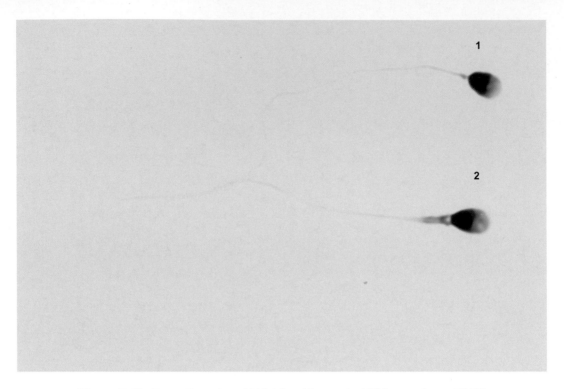

Figure 7.13: Rose Bengal and Toluidine blue stain (Oil immersion × 5000)

Number 1: This oval sperm head with normal acrosome measures 4.6 µm in length and 3.7 µm in width. The length to the width ratio is 1.24 which is lesser than 1.5 and hence this borderline sperm head has to be classified as "amorphous".

Number 2: An elongated sperm head measures 5.5 µm in length and 3.5 µm in width. The length to the width ratio is 1.57 which is normal. The WHO Manual (1999) states that the sperm head should measure 4 to 5 µm in length. In this case the elongated sperm head exceeds 5 µm in length. Hence, it is classified as a "Large" sperm head because the size of the sperm head takes precedence over the shape in morphology classification. Two distinct midpieces are discernible. The two tails are fused together.

A LARGE SPERM HEAD

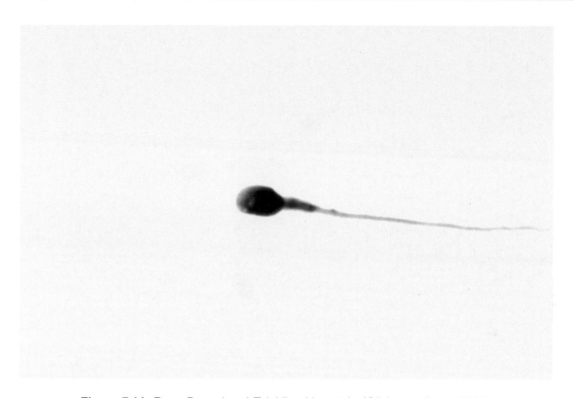

Figure 7.14: Rose Bengal and Toluidine blue stain (Oil immersion × 5000)

This picture illustrates a spermatozoon with large head. The sperm head measures 5.63 μm in length and 4.16 μm in width. The length to a width ratio is 1.35. The acrosome is small and slanting. There is asymmetry of the post acrosomal portion of the nucleus. The midpiece is thickened as it measures 1.96 μm in thickness. The tail is normal. Two nuclear vacuoles (stained pink) are seen at the junction of acrosome and the nucleus.

The large sperm heads are often associated with other defects either of acrosomes, midpieces or tails. Therefore, the fertility potential of megalosperms is supposedly reduced.

SMALL SPERM HEADS

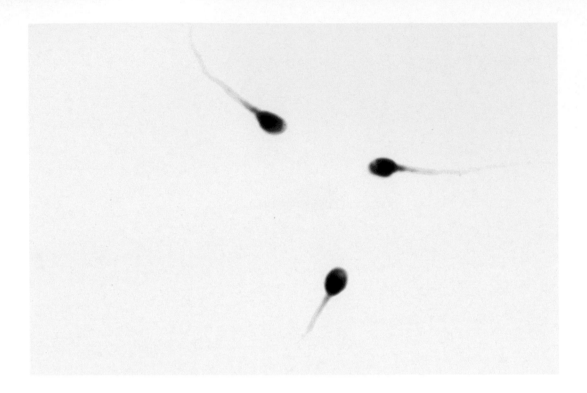

Figure 7.15: Rose Bengal and Toluidine blue stain (Oil immersion × 5000)

This picture illustrates the small sperm heads. Their average length is 3.53 µm and their average width is 2.74 µm. Such spermatozoa are classified as "Microsperms." It should be noted that only those sperm heads that are oval in shape but smaller in size are included in this category. Not only such spermatozoa may have acrosomal, midpiece and tail defects but also they often mimic the other sperm head abnormalities like "pyriform," "duplicate," "round" and "elongated type."

Increased percentage of microsperms in semen was the most statistically significant single sperm abnormality when pregnancy in vivo did not occur (Jauannet et al., 1988).

A TAPERED SPERM HEAD

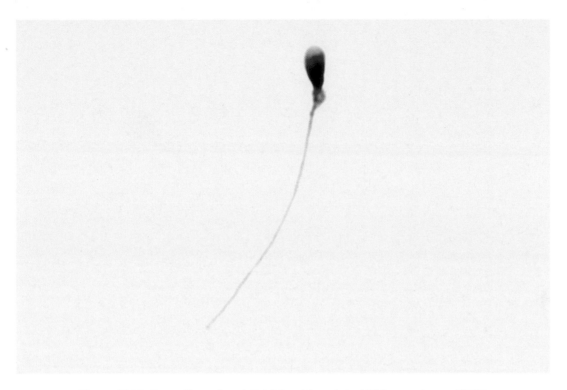

Figure 7.16: Rose Bengal and Toluidine blue stain (Oil immersion × 5000)

The 'Tapered' sperm heads are not to be confused with other sperm heads which are "Flame shaped" or resemble "Arrow heads." These latter sperm heads are to be included in the "amorphous" category. This picture illustrates a sperm with tapered head. The cytoplasmic extrusion mass attached to the otherwise normal midpiece is to be considered as normal. The tail is short and thick.

The typical 'tapered' sperm head is "cigar" shaped. Such sperms may compete with normal spermatozoa in ovum penetration. Since a normal pro-nucleus formation is unlikely in this situation, such spermatozoa should be considered as abnormal (Bartoov et al., 1982).

The tapered sperm heads assume a narrowed form due to the flattening of their sides. They are associated with varicoceles and bacterial infections (Zaneveld and Polakashi 1977).

A PYRIFORM SPERM HEAD

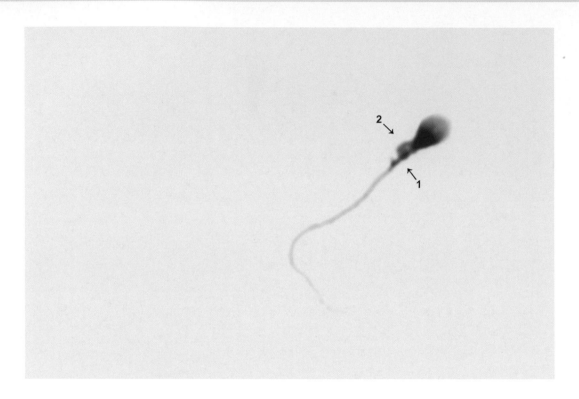

Figure 7.17: Rose Bengal and Toluidine blue stain (Oil immersion × 5000)

Unlike WHO classification of sperm morphology (1999) which has accorded a special identity to the "Pyriform heads" under the category of "Head defects," Tygerberg classification of sperm morphology has not accorded any special identity to the "Pyriform heads."

Pyriform sperm heads are identified due to their sharp pointed post-acrosomal base region. This abnormality is related to infertility. In the mammals the increased percentage of such forms in their ejaculates is associated with infertility.

The pyriform sperm heads, though may have width greater than 3.5 µm, should not be classified as "Large sperm heads." The shape of the sperm head rather than its size is the deciding factor.

The sperm depicted here has a pyriform head with normal acrosome, and an irregular midpiece (Arrow 1) but the tail is normal. The cytoplasmic extrusion mass attached to the midpiece (Arrow 2) should be considered as normal because its size is lesser than one-third the size of the sperm head.

ROUND HEADED SPERMATOZOA

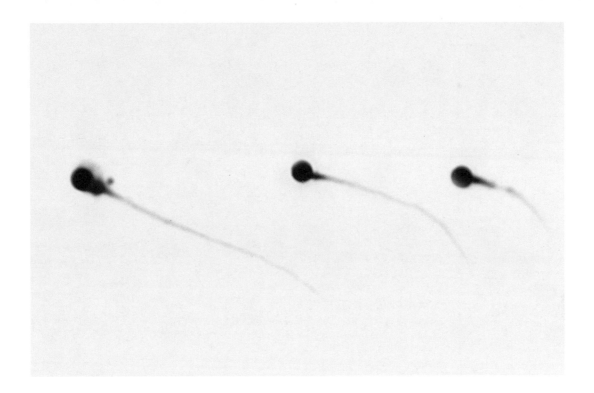

Figure 7.18: Rose Bengal and Toluidine blue stain (Oil immersion × 5000)

The "Round headed " spermatozoa are of two types namely, "Round headed" spermatozoa with acrosomes and "Small round headed " spermatozoa without acrosomes.

This picture illustrates the small round headed spermatozoa without acrosomes. This round headed sperm defect is described as "Globozoospermia" and constitutes the best example of " specific sterilizing defects" in humans. For the further description of this lesion please also refer to the next figure.

These small round headed spermatozoa can be double headed or triple headed. Such sperms can also have double or multiple tails.

Infertile men having 'Globozoospermia' are incurable and can father a child through the assisted reproductive techniques such as I.C.S.I.

ROUND HEADED SPERMATOZOA WITHOUT ACROSOMES

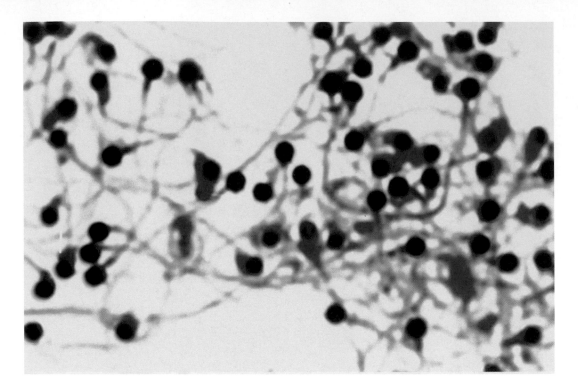

Figure 7.19: Rose Bengal and Toluidine blue stain (Oil immersion × 5000)

The round headed spermatozoa are subdivided into two categories. (1) Round headed spermatozoa with acrosomes and (2) Round headed spermatozoa without acrosomes.

This small round head defect is described as "globozoospermia" and constitutes the best-known example of specific sterilizing defects in humans. Failure of acrosomes to develop is ascribed as an etiological factor.

However, ultrastructure studies of testicular biopsies obtained from infertile men having globozoospermia, have demonstrated that acrosomal vesicle is frequent in young spermatids. (Holstein et al., 1973 and Baccetti et al., 1977). Further development of vesicles does not take place. After spermiation the vesicles that are left behind are digested by Sertoli cells.

SPERMATOZOA WITH ROUND HEADS

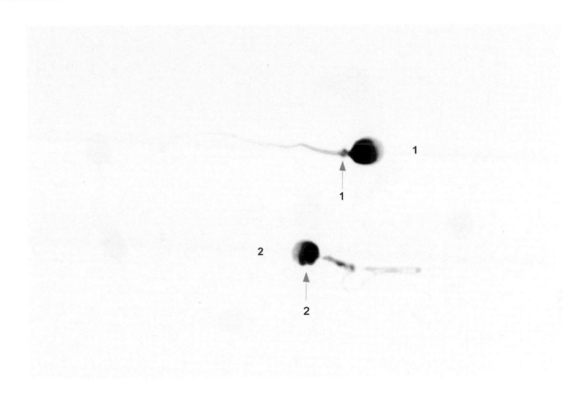

Figure 7.20: Rose Bengal and Toluidine blue stain (Oil immersion × 5000)

Number 1: This picture illustrates a round headed spermatozoon with normal acrosome. A cytoplasmic twig attached to the midpiece (Arrow 1) that is otherwise normal, is to be considered as normal. The tail is normal. The sperm head measures 4.6 μm in length and 3 μm in width. The length to the width ratio is 1.53

Number 2: The round head of this sperm measures 2.9 μm in length and 3.3 μm in width. The length to the width ratio is 1.26. On the inferior margin of the post acrosomal portion of the nucleus, a vacuole can be identified (Arrow 2). The midpiece is thickened and the tail is looped.

The round nucleus of the sperm head probably indicates a failure of the nuclear transformation during spermiogenesis.

AMORPHOUS SPERMATOZOA

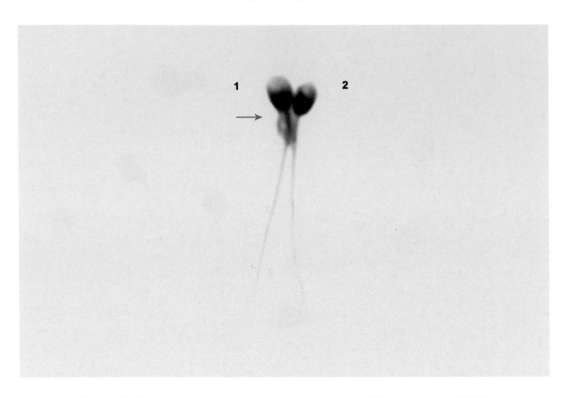

Figure 7.23: Rose Bengal and Toluidine blue stain (Oil immersion × 5000)

This picture illustrates a duplicate or conjoined form.

Number 1:   A spermatozoon with normal head and acrosome, has a thickened midpiece but its tail is normal.

Number 2:   A microsperm with a small acrosome has an indistinct midpiece but has a normal tail. A cytoplasmic extrusion mass (Arrow), is holding together parts of sperm heads and midpieces.

In the duplicate forms the site of fusion could either be at the head, midpiece or tail region.

AMORPHOUS SPERMATOZOA

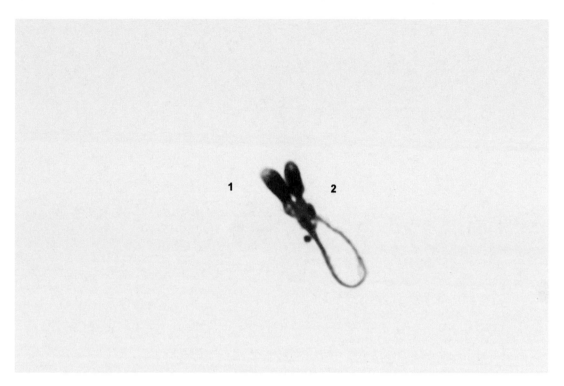

Figure 7.24: Rose Bengal and Toluidine blue stain (Oil immersion × 5000)

There is no special subgroup for "Duplicate forms" listed under the category of "Sperm head defects" in the twin systems of sperm morphology classifications, either of WHO or of Tygerberg.

The "duplicate form" is the result of fusion or incomplete separation of two sperms either at head, midpiece or tail region.

In this picture the tails of two spermatozoa are fused together. In addition to this, the constituent spermatozoa are adherent together at the midpiece region.

Sperm head Number 1: This sperm has an elongated head and a thickening of the lower portion of its midpiece. The tail is fused together with the tail of its counterpart.

Sperm head Number 2: A sperm with amorphous head and small acrosome has a thickening of the lower portion of its midpiece. The tail of each sperm is fused with the tail of its counterpart.

A TRINUCLEATE SPERM HEAD

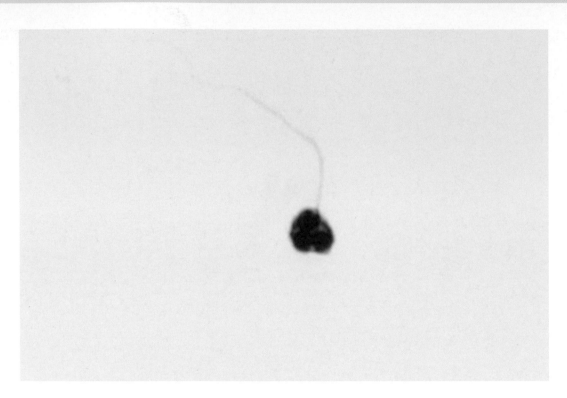

Figure 7.25: Rose Bengal and Toluidine blue stain (Oil immersion × 5000)

A trinucleate sperm head is depicted here. This patient had "Globozoospermia". Note that the three round nuclei of the sperm are enclosed in the cytoplasm. The midpiece is not discernible. The tail is normal.

This type of the sperm head is not to be confused with multicephalic sperm head observed in the same patient. See Figure 7.26 on the next page.

AMORPHOUS AND OTHER SPERM HEADS

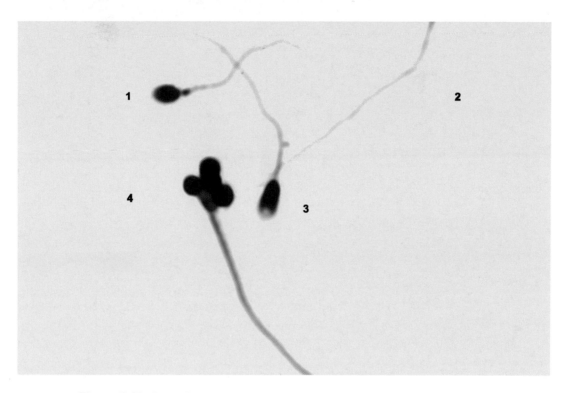

Figure 7.26: Rose Bengal and Toluidine blue stain (Oil immersion × 5000)

Number 1: A microsperm with a small acrosome has a small midpiece and its tail is thickened.

Number 2: A "pin headed" sperm.

Number 3: This sperm has an elongated head with a small acrosome and though its midpiece is normal the tail is thick and short.

Number 4: Note that this spermatozoon has four round heads without acrososomes. The sperm heads are as if implanted in a cytoplasmic mass in the neck region, from which a single thick tail has emerged. This quadricephalic sperm head is not to be confused with multinucleate sperm head.

AMORPHOUS SPERM HEADS

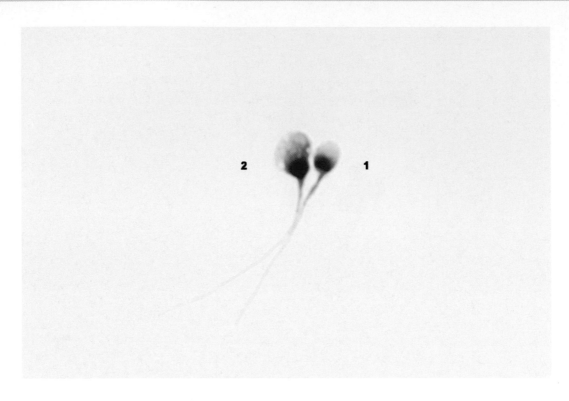

Figure 7.27: Rose Bengal and Toluidine blue stain (Oil immersion × 5000)

Number 1: An amorphous sperm head has normal acrosome. The midpiece that is attached slightly ab-axially is otherwise normal. The tail is normal.

Number 2: A large non-oval amorphous sperm head has a large acrosome covering 80 percent of the head area. The mega acrosome shows the presence of three distinct pale stained vacuoles. The midpiece, attached ab-axially, is normal. The tail is normal.

A TRICEPHALIC SPERM HEAD

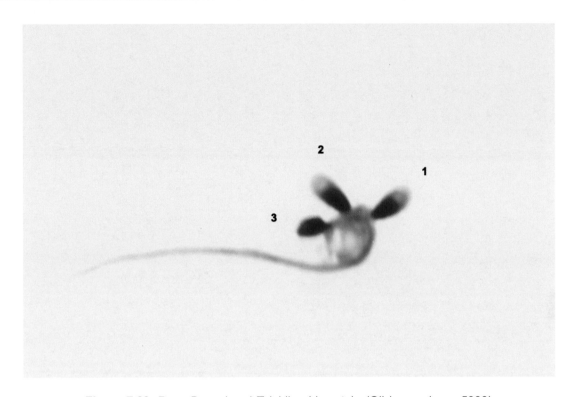

Figure 7.28: Rose Bengal and Toluidine blue stain (Oil immersion × 5000)

A pleomorphic (amorphous) sperm has a tricephalic sperm head. The sperm heads (Number 1 and 2) are elongated but have normal acrosomes. The third head (Number 3) is deformed and has no acrosome.

There is a large vacuolated cytoplasmic extrusion mass at the midpiece region. The midpieces of the individual sperms are not discernible. Their common thickened midpiece and a common thick tail is seen emerging out from the cytoplasmic mass.

Such multicephalic forms owe their origin possibly to multinucleate spermatids.

A MULTICEPHALIC AMORPHOUS HEAD

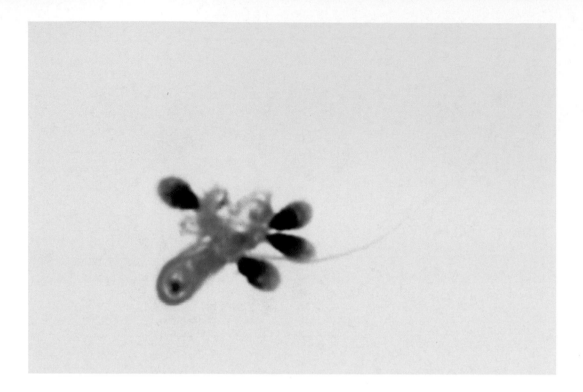

Figure 7.29: Rose Bengal and Toluidine blue stain (Oil immersion × 5000)

An amorphous spermatozoon with four elongated heads is depicted here. The sperm heads, that show normal acrosomes are as if implanted in a huge spanner shaped cytoplasmic mass. Few tails are seen entangled in the cytoplasmic mass. One faint tail is seen emerging out on the right side. The individual midpieces are not identifiable.

AN AMORPHOUS SPERM

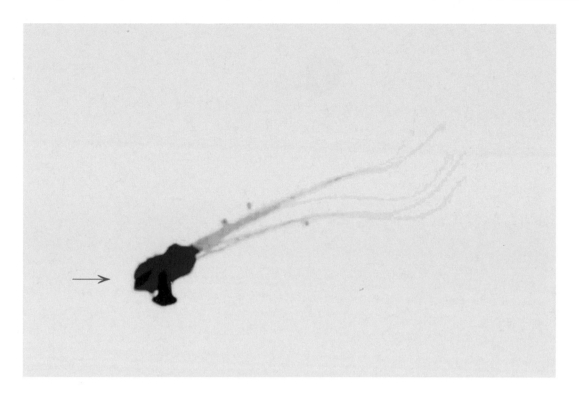

Figure 7.30: Rose Bengal and Toluidine blue stain (Oil immersion × 5000)

The varieties of amorphous forms are legion. In this picture note that the flattened sperm head is without an acrosome. It has a thick long neck that is connected to a veritable broom of tails. There is a large cytoplasmic mass in place of the midpiece from which five distinct tails are emerging on the right side. Another head like structure (Arrow) is seen in the cytoplasmic mass.

AN AMORPHOUS SPERM

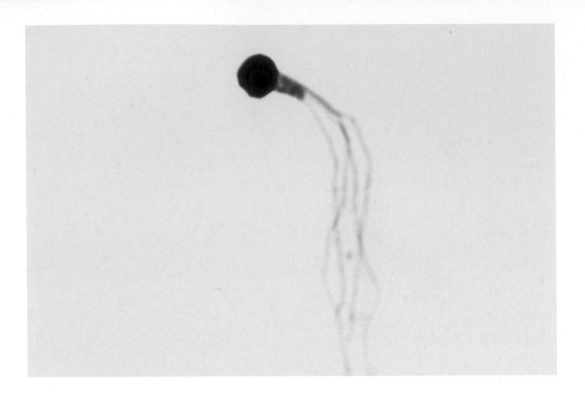

Figure 7.31: Rose Bengal and Toluidine blue stain (Oil immersion × 5000)

This picture illustrates an amorphous sperm. The sperm head, though large, should not be classified as "Large sperm head" because it is abnormal. Note that the giant round head has no acrosome. The midpiece is thickened. From the midpiece four distinct tails are seen emerging out and going downwards.

This sperm has "Multiple sperm abnormalities." The sperm head that is large and round in shape is devoid of an acrosome. The midpiece is thickened and there are multiple tails.

A BIZARRE AMORPHOUS SPERM

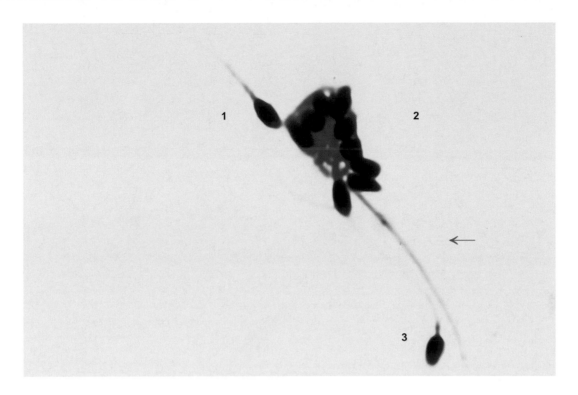

Figure 7.32: Rose Bengal and Toluidine blue stain (Oil immersion × 5000)

Number 1: Note that this elongated microsperm has a small acrosome but the midpiece and tail are normal.

Number 2: A bizarre amorphous sperm is illustrated here. Note that a group of ten sperm heads, devoid of acrosomes, is engulfed in a cytoplasmic mass formed by the intermixing of tails. One thick tail (Arrow) is seen emanating downwards from the network of tails. This form should not be confused with a "Multinucleate sperm head" because there is an absence of the cell cytoplasm surrounding the ten distinct sperm heads.

Number 3: An elongated microsperm with absence of an acrosome has a short midpiece but its tail is normal.

AN ELONGATED SPERM HEAD

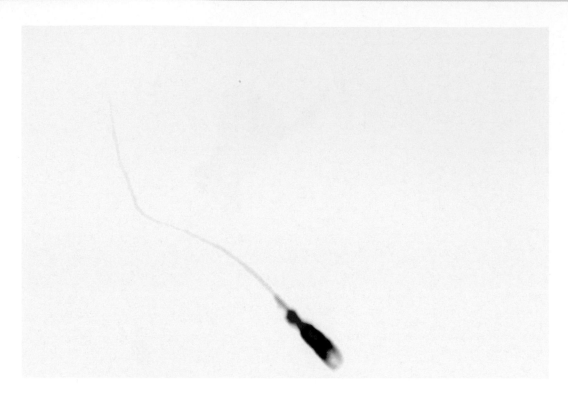

Figure 7.33: Rose Bengal and Toluidine blue stain (Oil immersion × 5000)

Unlike the WHO classification of sperm morphology, the Tygerberg classification has a subgroup of "Elongated heads" listed under sperm head defects.

This sperm head, with almost equal distribution of acrosomal and post-acrosomal areas, measures 5.5 µm in length and has a width of 1.8 µm. According to Düsseldorf classification (1985, 1987–refer Hoffman and Haider 1985 and Hoffman et al., 1987) it would be classified as "Type HI°" defect. The sperm heads, with equal distribution of acrosomal and post-acrosomal areas, exceeding 5 µm in length and with a width lesser than 3.5 µm are included in this category.

Elongated spermatozoa not only are capable of penetrating and migrating through the cervical mucus, (Fredicsson and Bjork, 1977; Mortimer, D. et al., 1982) but are also capable of binding with zona pellucida. (Menkweld, R 1991; Liu and Baker 1992).

This aberration is thought to be due to functional disorders of Sertoli cells and environmental factors, and is considered to be reversible.

AN AMORPHOUS AND A TAPERED SPERM HEAD

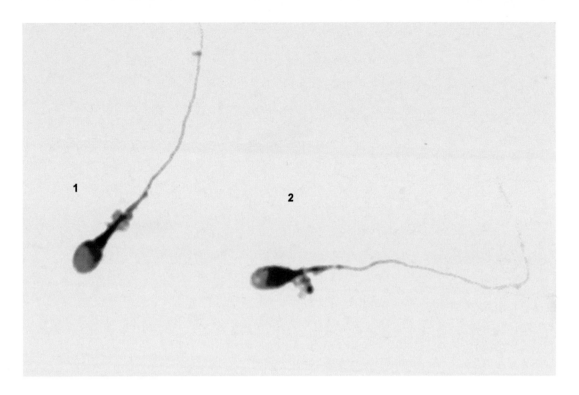

Figure 7.34: Rose Bengal and Toluidine blue stain (Oil immersion × 5000)

WHO classification of sperm morphology (1999) enlists tapered sperm heads as a separate entity under the "Sperm head defects." In Tygerberg classification, "Tapered" and "Elongated sperm heads," are clubbed together under "Sperm head defects."

Number 1: This sperm head has a cone shaped elongation of the post-acrosomal portion of the nucleus. This differentiates it from "Pyriform head." As per Düsseldorf's classification (1985 and 1987 – refer Hoffman and Haider 1985 and Hoffman et al., 1987) this defect is to be listed as "Type H-II°" defect. This abnormality is due to a Sertoli cell dysfunction and is considered to be reversible.

Number 2: A "Tapered" sperm head has a "Cigar shaped" appearance due to flattening of the sides. Such tapered heads are not to be confused with "Flame shaped" heads that are tapered anteriorly. Increased percentage of spermatozoa with tapered heads is associated with varicoceles and bacterial infections (Zanveld and Polsakashi 1977).

ELONGATED SPERM HEADS

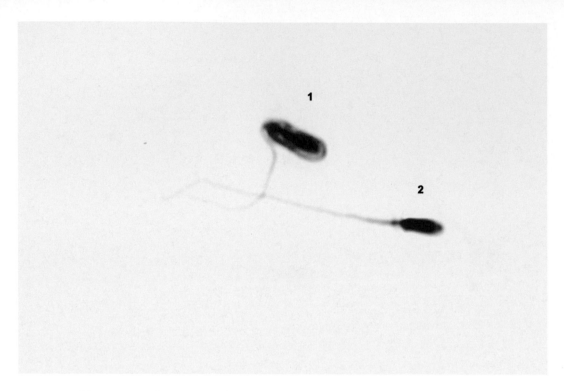

Figure 7.35: Rose Bengal and Toluidine blue stain (Oil immersion × 5000)

Unlike the Tygerberg classification of sperm morphology, the WHO classification (1999) does not have a separate subcategory of "Elongated heads" listed under sperm head defects. However the Tygerberg's classification clubs together three abnormal forms of sperm heads like "Pyriform heads," "Tapered heads" and "Elongated heads" in this subcategory.

Number 1: This sperm head, with an absence of acrosome, has a severe and extensive elongation of the nucleus ending in a button like formation. According to Düsseldorf classification 1985, 1987 – refer Hoffman and Haider 1985 and Hoffman 1987), this type of defect is irreversible and is classified as " H III°" defect. The midpiece is bent and the tail is seen coiling around the head (surrounded by cytoplasm) before unwinding. This constitutes a severe form of "Dag defect ".

Number 2: An elongated sperm head, with a short acrosome, has a normal midpiece and tail.

A DUMBBELL SHAPED SPERM HEAD

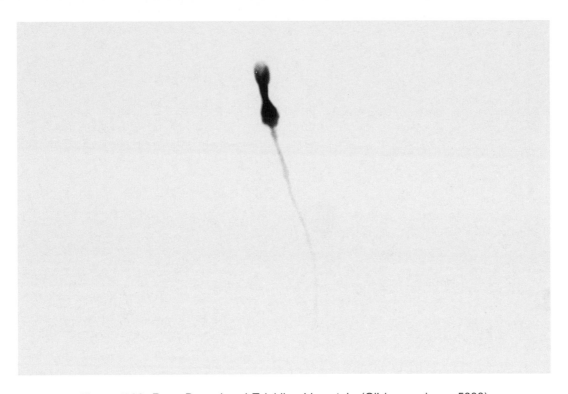

Figure 7.36: Rose Bengal and Toluidine blue stain (Oil immersion × 5000)

This picture illustrates a "dumbbell" shaped sperm head. It measures 8.37 µm in length and has a maximum width of 2.84 µm. The sperm head has a small acrosome. The post-acrosomal portion of the nucleus exhibits an extreme elongation and ends in a button like a knob. The midpiece and the tail are normal.

According to Düsseldorf classification (1985, 1987 – refer Hoffman and Haider 1985, Hoffman 1987) this type of defect is irreversible and is classified as "H III°" defect. It is believed that this type of defect is due to the dysfunction of Sertoli cells.

Unlike the Tygerberg classification of sperm morphology, the WHO classification of sperm morphology (1999) does not have a separate entity of "Elongated heads" listed under sperm head defects.

INCOMPLETE DUPLICATION

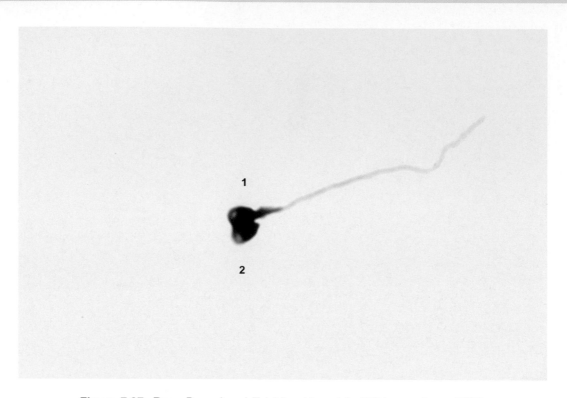

Figure 7.37: Rose Bengal and Toluidine blue stain (Oil immersion × 5000)

This picture illustrates a microsperm (No. 1). It has a small acrosome, thick neck, a normal midpiece and tail. An accessory sperm head (No. 2) is laterally adherent to the original sperm head. However, this accessory sperm head is devoid of a midpiece and tail.

Such forms indicate incomplete duplication. One can postulate their origin as follows. These forms owe their origin to binucleate spermatids whose nuclei are not separated completely. One of the spermatid nucleus has undergone spermiogenesis to produce a microsperm (No. 1). The other incompletely separated spermatid nucleus shows arrested development during spermiogenesis in as much as the midpiece and tail are not developed.

Similar adherent extra sperm heads are sometimes associated with duplicate and triplicate forms.

NORMAL AND AMORPHOUS SPERMATOZOA

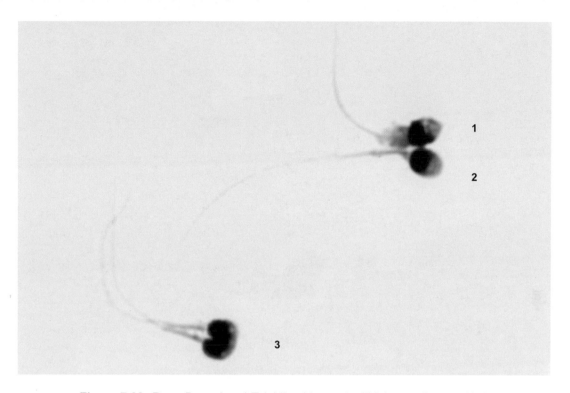

Figure 7.38: Rose Bengal and Toluidine blue stain (Oil immersion × 5000)

Number 1:   An amorphous sperm head has irregular edges and a ragged acrosome. The midpiece is surrounded by an irregular cytoplasmic extrusion mass but the tail is normal.

Number 2:   A normal sperm with a normal head, acrosome, midpiece and tail.

Number 3:   A terratoid (amorphous) sperm is depicted here. There are three heads, with normal acrosomes, that are adhering laterally to each other. The sperm head at the top and the other at the bottom have their own distinct midpieces and tails. The extra sperm head that is sandwiched between the upper and lower sperm head is devoid of its own midpiece or a tail.

ABNORMAL SPERM HEADS

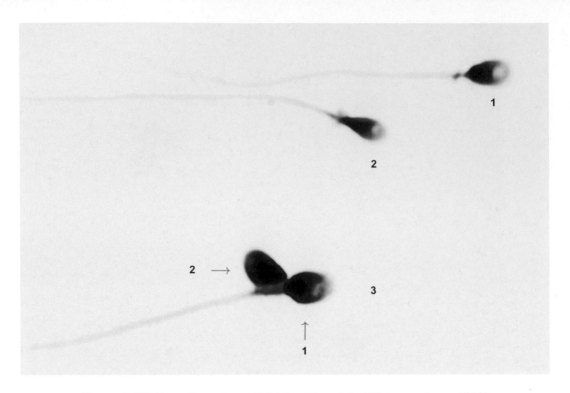

Figure 7.39: Rose Bengal and Toluidine blue stain (Oil immersion × 5000)

Number 1: This sperm has an elongated head with a normal acrosome, a short midpiece and a normal tail.

Number 2: Tapered sperm head with a normal acrosome has a cytoplasmic twig attached to the midpiece. The tail is normal.

Number 3: This megalosperm has a giant head (Arrow 1) but the midpiece and tail are normal. An accessory head (Arrow 2), with a small acrosome is attached laterally to the midpiece of the megalosperm by means of a membranous adhesion. This abnormal sperm should not be confused with a true double headed sperm.

ABNORMAL SPERMATOZOA

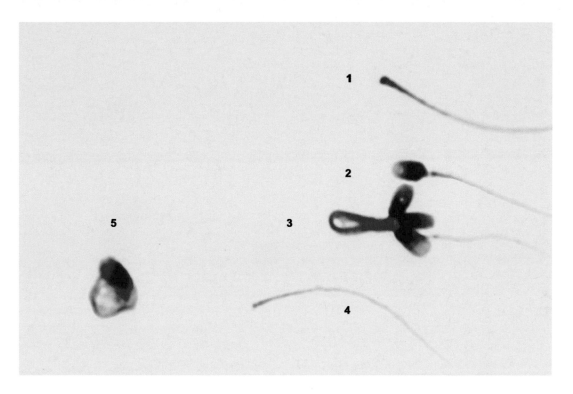

Figure 7.40: Rose Bengal and Toluidine blue stain (Oil immersion × 5000)

Number 1: and Number 4: The pin-headed spermatozoa.

Number 2: This sperm has an elongated head with a normal acrosome, and a normal midpiece and tail.

Number 3: This picture shows a tricephalic sperm that has three elongated heads with normal acrosomes. It shows fusion of at least of two midpieces. The tails of these two constituent sperms are fused together and looped. The tail of one sperm has formed a loop before emerging out.

Number 5: This tapered sperm head has a normal acrosome. The tail is curled around the midpiece and around a vacuolated cytoplasmic mass. This illustrates the so called "Dag defect."

NUCLEAR VACUOLES AND MEGA ACROSOME

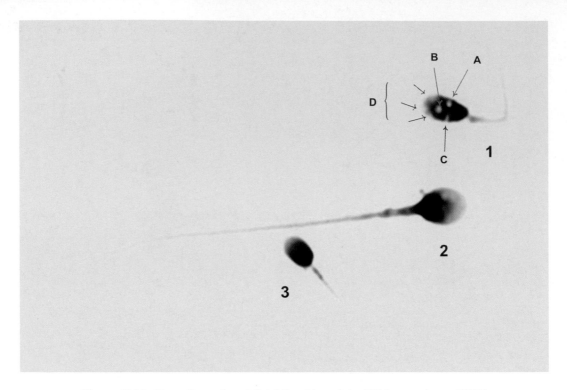

Figure 7.41: Rose Bengal and Toluidine blue stain (Oil immersion × 5000)

Number 1: An amorphous sperm head shows the presence of two nuclear vacuoles, marked as, "A" and "B". The vacuole "B" is at the equatorial region. The lower margin of the nucleus shows the presence of a cytoplasmic invagination into the nucleus that is marked as "C". Few faint stained acrosomal vacuoles are marked as "D". The midpiece is small. The tail is bent.

Number 2: A large pyriform sperm head has a mega-acrosome. The midpiece and tail are thickened.

Number 3: A microsperm has a normal acrosome but the midpiece is small and the tail is indistinct.

NUCLEAR VACUOLES WITH DIADEM DEFECT

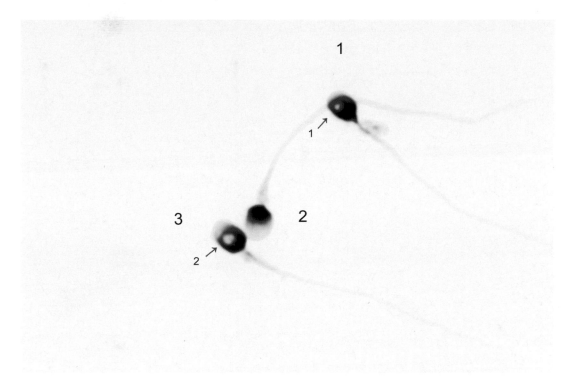

Figure 7.42: Rose Bengal and Toluidine blue stain (Oil immersion × 5000)

Number 1: An amorphous sperm head with a small acrosome shows a nuclear vacuole (Arrow 1) at the equatorial region. The midpiece shows attached cytoplasm.

Number 2: This amorphous sperm head has a normal acrosome.

Number 3: An amorphous sperm head has an equatorial vacuole (Arrow 2). This vacuole as vacuole number 1, has a pale center with a dark perimeter. Both such vacuoles usually are not empty and when seen in a row at the equatorial region resemble a "diadem," meaning a crown. Note that such diadem vacuoles are the result of a single or multiple cytoplasmic invaginations into the nucleus and are usually at the equatorial region. The diadem vacuoles are discrete and may contain remnants of cytoplasmic material.

DUPLICATE, TAPERED AND DEFECTIVE SPERM HEADS

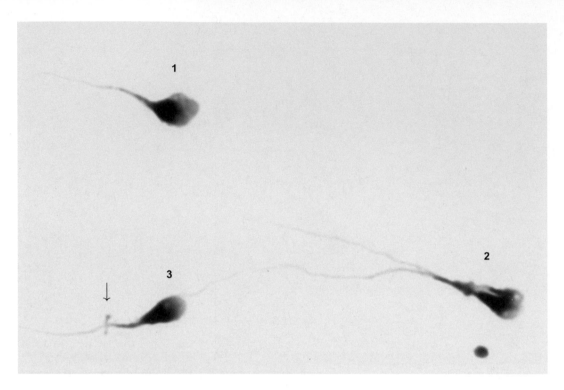

Figure 7.43: Rose Bengal and Toluidine blue stain (Oil immersion × 5000)

Number 1: An amorphous sperm head has an irregular acrosome. The post-acrosomal portion of the nucleus, midpiece and tail are normal.

Number 2: A duplicate form shows that the two spermatozoa with elongated heads are attached to each other at the region of their heads and midpieces. The midpiece of the lower sperm is thickened. Two separate tails are easily identifiable.

Number 3: A sperm with a tapered head with normal acrosome has a normal midpiece. An intersecting bar (Arrow) is seen at the region of the annulus. This is a frequent finding.

SPERM HEAD WITH BASAL NUCLEAR VACUOLES

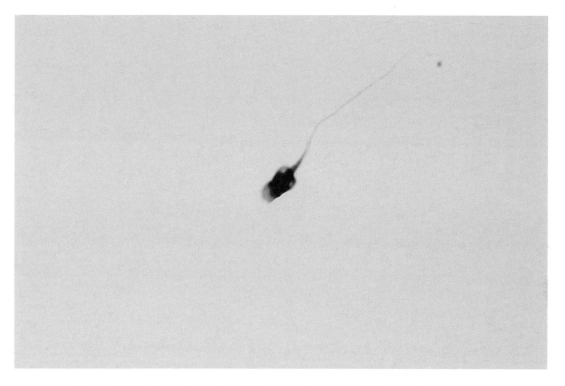

Figure 7.44: Rose Bengal and Toluidine blue stain (Oil immersion × 5000)

An elongated sperm head shows two basal nuclear vacuoles. The presence of these vacuoles has distorted the shape of the basal part of the nucleus. The protuberant acrosomal cap is distinct. The midpiece and tail are normal.

Normally the nuclear vacuoles vary in size and as a rule they are empty. However, the diadem defect vacuoles are always membrane lined due to the cytoplasmic invagination into the nucleus. The vacuoles illustrated above are due to areas of defective condensation in the nucleus and do not represent diadem defect.

NUCLEAR INVAGINATION AND NUCLEAR VACUOLE

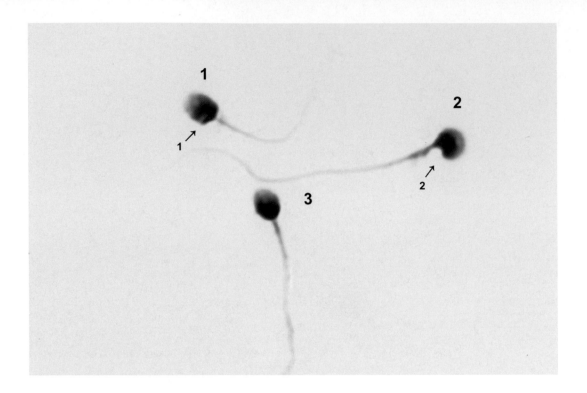

Figure 7.45: Rose Bengal and Toluidine blue stain (Oil immersion × 5000)

Number 1: An amorphous sperm head has an abnormal length to a width ratio. At the inferior margin of the nucleus there is a cytoplasmic invagination (Arrow 1).

Number 2: A basal nuclear vacuole (Arrow 2) has distorted the shape of the post-acrosomal portion of the nucleus. The midpiece attachment is ab-axial but the tail is normal.

Number 3: A normal sperm head has a slightly ab-axial attachment of the midpiece. The tail is thickened.

BORDERLINE AND TERATOID SPERMATOZOA

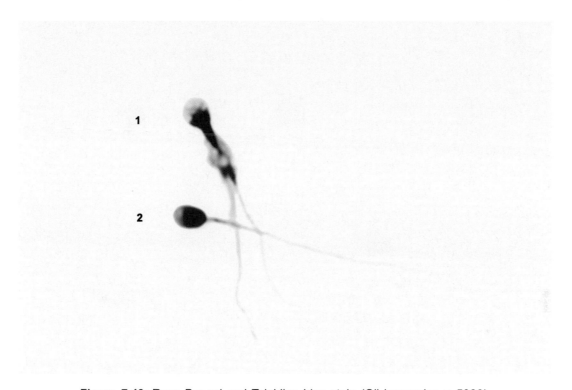

Figure 7.46: Rose Bengal and Toluidine blue stain (Oil immersion × 5000)

Number 1: This spermatozoon has multiple defects. The sperm head, measuring 9.1 µm in length, shows a stalk like elongation of the post-acrosomal portion of the nucleus. This type of defect is classified as "Type H-II°" defect in Düsseldorf's classification (1985, 1987 – refer Hoffman and Haider 1985, Hoffman et al., Hoffman 1987). WHO classification of sperm morphology (1999) does not have a separate category, under "head defects" for elongated sperm heads. The sperm head is also to be classified as "vacuolated" as more than 20% of the head area is occupied by vacuoles (WHO 1999). There is circular cytoplasmic extrusion mass surrounding the two midpieces. It also has two tails.

Number 2: A near normal borderline form is to be considered abnormal. The sperm head measures 3.8 µm in length and 2.7 µm in width. The length to a width ratio is 1.4. The acrosome is small. The midpiece and tail are normal.

NORMAL AND ABNORMAL SPERMATOZOA

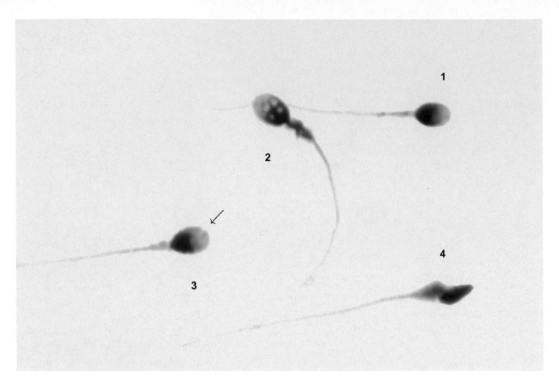

Figure 7.47: Rose Bengal and Toluidine blue stain (Oil immersion × 5000)

Number 1: This sperm has a normal head, acrosome, midpiece and a normal tail.

Number 2: This sperm has a large head that shows four vacuoles, two in the acrosomal portion of the nucleus and two in the nuclear region. The thickened and tortuous midpiece is inserted asymmetrically into the sperm head. The tail is thick.

Number 3: A large sperm head has an acrosomal vacuole (Arrow). The midpiece is not well defined.

Number 4: A small flame shaped sperm head is devoid of acrosome. The thickened midpiece is inserted asymmetrically into the sperm head.

A VACUOLATED SPERM HEAD

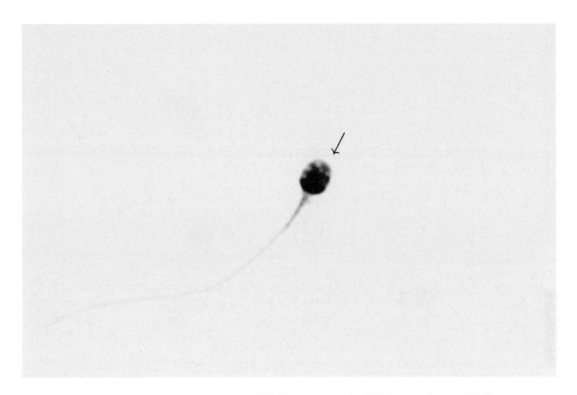

Figure 7.48: Rose Bengal and Toluidine blue stain (Oil immersion × 5000)

According to WHO classification of sperm morphology (1999), a sperm head is to be classified as "vacuolated" if more than 20% of the head area is occupied by vacuoles. Several sperm nuclei, commonly, have areas of incomplete condensation. These areas appear as vacuoles. Nuclear vacuoles are commonly found in the acrosomal portion of the sperm head. Thus, these areas of incomplete nuclear condensation are covered by acrosome and hence appear indistinct. However, vacuoles are also found in the post-acrosomal portion of the nucleus. The size of the nuclear vacuoles is variable. The presence of one to three nuclear vacuoles is to be considered as normal.

In this instance the sperm head is to be classified as ' vacuolated' and most of the vacuoles, if not all, are in the acrosomal region (Arrow).

Other than a vacuolated head, this sperm has a normal midpiece and a normal tail.

A CYTOPLASMIC HOOD COVERING THE SPERM HEAD

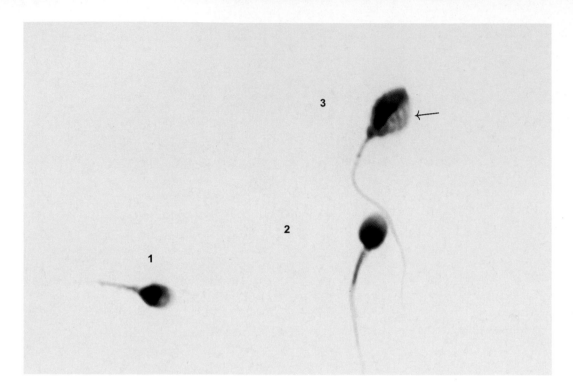

Figure 7.49: Rose Bengal and Toluidine blue stain (Oil immersion × 5000)

Number 1: The picture illustrates a normal sperm that has a normal head and acrosome. The post-acrosomal portion of the nucleus, though slightly tapered, is to be considered normal. The midpiece is thin. The tail is normal but indistinct.

Number 2: This picture depicts a normal sperm head with a normal acrosome. A slight asymmetry of the post-acrosomal portion of the nucleus is permissible. The midpiece and tail are normal.

Number 3: This picture depicts a tapered sperm head with a normal acrosome. A cytoplasmic shell (Arrow) is partially covering the nucleus. The midpiece and tail are normal.

A DOUBLE HEADED SPERM

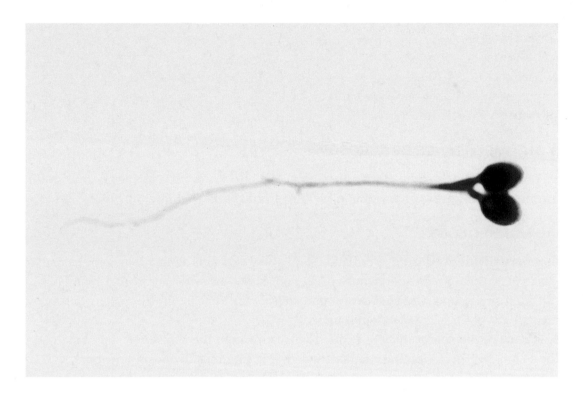

Figure 7.50: Rose Bengal and Toluidine blue stain (Oil immersion × 5000)

This picture illustrates a double headed sperm. Such forms should not be confused with the following abnormalities.

1. Additional sperm head attached laterally to the head of a sperm.
2. Binucleate sperm head with a single midpiece and tail.
3. Paired spermatozoa (Duplicate forms) with a conjoint segment at the midpiece or tail region.
4. Two bipolar sperm heads with an end to end fusion of tails.
5. Two distinct sperm's heads with a "U" shaped fusion of tails.

Double headed spermatozoa are incapable of fertilization and are more typical of a varicocele than of infectious diseases (MacLeod 1970: David et al., 1972)

2-B ABNORMALITIES OF SPERM ACROSOMES ADDENDUM

- Discovery and importance of acrosome.
- Acrosomal morphology.
- Biochemical aspects.
- Functional aspects.
- Acrosomal abnormalities as a separate entity.
- Acrosomal status Vis-á-vis infertility.

DISCOVERY AND IMPORTANCE OF ACROSOME

Williams (1934) described acrosome for the first time. We also know that the acrosomal status is the most important criterion for the predictive value in in vitro fertilization (Jeulin et al., 1986).

ACROSOMAL MORPHOLOGY

An acrosome is partially derived from spermatid Golgi apparatus. It is a bilaminar semi-transparent structure that covers 40 to 70% area of the sperm nucleus. It consists of an outer acrosomal membrane that lies just inside the cell membrane and an inner acrosomal membrane that is abutting the nuclear membrane. In between these two layers lies the acrosomal matrix.

The inner contour of the sperm nucleus is often visible through the acrosomal cap in stained preparations of semen. The Eosin-Nigrosin staining method reveals the fine meshwork of acrosome.

BIOCHEMICAL ASPECTS

An acrosome is a specialized lysosome and contains several hydrolytic enzymes like hyaluradinase, protease, acid phosphatase and pro-acrosin which are necessary for fertilization.

FUNCTIONAL ASPECTS

Acrosome is essential for fertilization. Fusion of the outer acrosomal membrane (acrosomal reaction) releases lytic enzymes. The outer cell membrane and the outer acrosomal membrane undergoes dissolution. The nuclear membrane and the inner acrosomal membrane then surround the acrosomal part of the nucleus. The equatorial region segment of acrosomal region, is the initial region of sperm egg fusion.

ACROSOMAL ABNORMALITIES AS A SEPARATE ENTITY

An acrosomal abnormality as a separate entity, under the category of "Sperm head defects," was included in their sperm morphology classifications by Williams (1934) and Weisman (1941). This entity was ignored by the subsequent investigators and was lost in oblivion. It was resurrected after more than fifty years when WHO Manual (1999) incorporated "Acrosomal defects" as a separate subgroup under the category of "Sperm head defects."

However, WHO classification (1999) of sperm morphology has listed a solitary acrosomal abnormality, namely, short acrosomes, as a representative acrosomal defect under the category of "Sperm head defects". Nevertheless, the Manual emphasizes "Absence of acrosomes" while describing "Globozoospermia".

This Atlas includes several other photographs documenting important acrosomal lesions.

ACROSOMAL STATUS VIS-Á-VIS INFERTILITY

The causal relationship between the following acrosomal defects and infertility is well established.

1. Absence of acrosomes.
2. Patchy acrosomes.
3. Detached acrosomes.
4. Small acrosomes.
5. Acrosomal vacuoles.
6. Ruptured acrosomes.
7. Nipple acrosomes.
8. Acrosomal cysts.
9. Degenerating acrosomes.

Acrosomal defects whose effect on infertility is not known.

1. Mega acrosomes.
2. Deformed acrosomes.
3. Oversized acrosomes.
4. Multilocular acrosomes.
5. Lateral acrosomes.
6. Acrosomal invagination into the nucleus.

ACROSOMES OF ABNORMAL SPERMATOZOA

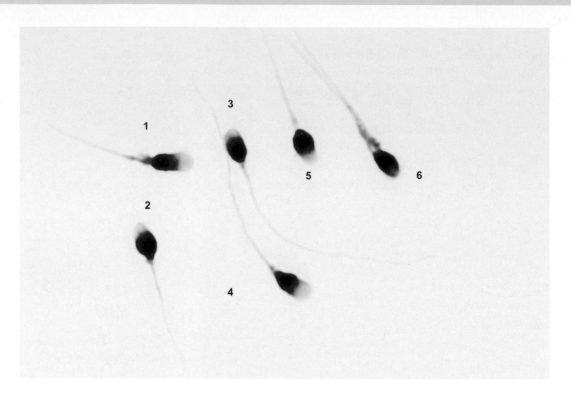

Figure 7.51: Rose Bengal and Toluidine blue stain (Oil immersion × 5000)

This picture illustrates acrosomes of abnormal spermatozoa. The acrosomes are stained pink. The junctions of acrosomes and sperm nuclei are sharply delineated. The post-acrosomal portions of sperm nuclei are stained deep blue. The midpieces and tails are stained pink.

Numbers 1,3 and 4:   These spermatozoa have elongated heads. The sperms, number 1 and 4 have a protuberance like acrosomes. The sperm number 3 has a normal acrosome.

Numbers 2, 5 and 6:   These pictures represent the microsperms. The sperms, number 2 and 5 have normal acrosomes. The sperm number 6 has a small acrosome, thick midpiece and a double tail.

SPERMATOZOA WITH SMALL ACROSOMES

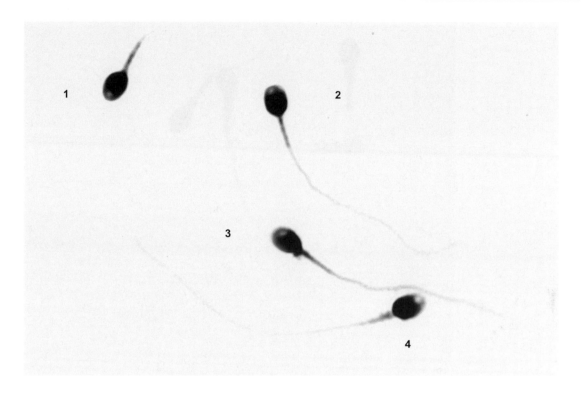

Figure 7.52: Rose Bengal and Toluidine blue stain (Oil immersion × 5000)

This picture illustrates microsperms with small acrosomes. However, their midpieces and tails are normal.

Number 1: The sperm head shows asymmetry of the post-acrosomal portion of the nucleus.

Number 2: The sperm head has a normal oval configuration.

Number 3: The sperm head is of a "pyriform" type.

Number 4: The sperm head is of an "elongated" type.

LARGE, HYPERTROPHIED AND SHORT ACROSOMES

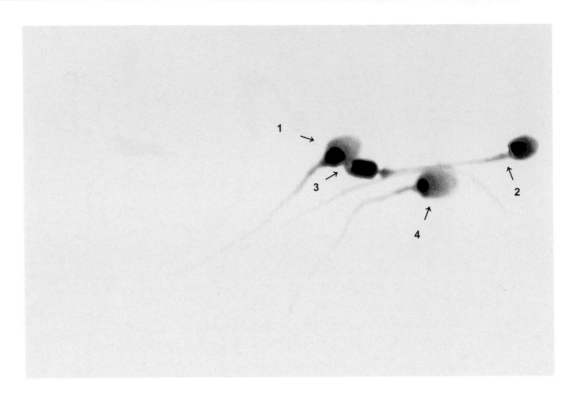

Figure 7.55: Rose Bengal and Toluidine blue stain (Oil immersion × 5000)

The

and h

Numb

Numb

Numb

Number 1: A tapered sperm head has a hypertrophied acrosome (Arrow 1). Note the asymmetry of the post-acrosomal portion of the nucleus.

Number 2: The sperm head of a microsperm has a small acrosome. The midpiece is asymmetrically inserted into the sperm head (Arrow 2). The tail is normal.

Number 3: An elongated sperm head has a short acrosome (Arrow 3).

Number 4: A large sperm head has a balloon shaped acrosome covering almost the entire head area (Arrow 4).

ACROSOMES OF AMORPHOUS SPERMATOZOA

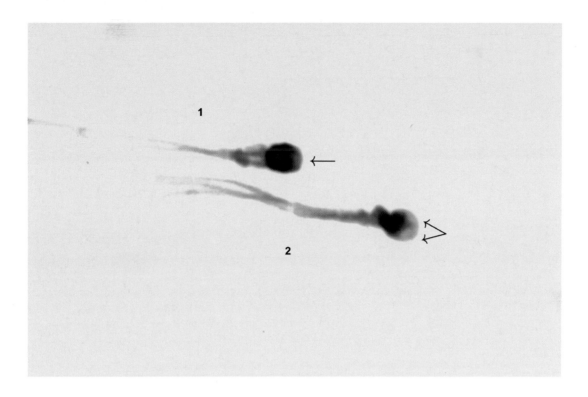

Figure 7.56: Rose Bengal and Toluidine blue stain (Oil immersion × 5000)

Number 1: A duplicate form is illustrated here. Note that the sperm heads of both the sperms are fused together. The two sperm heads have a common small acrosome (Arrow). The midpieces are normal and are engulfed in a common cytoplaspmic mass. The two emerging tails, which are fused at the beginning, are separated from each other distally.

Number 2: This double headed bizarre sperm shows fusion of two sperms at the head and midpiece region. Note that the two sperm heads have separate acrosomes (Twin arrows). The elongated fused midpieces are immersed in a mass of cytoplasm, from which three tails are emerging out.

SPERMATOZOA WITH LATERAL ACROSOMES

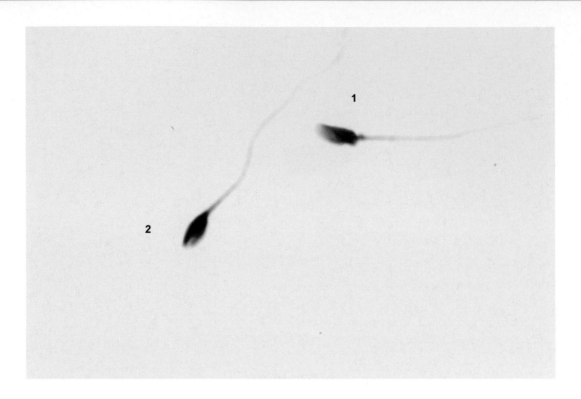

Figure 7.57: Rose Bengal and Toluidine blue stain (Oil immersion × 5000)

The spermatozoa depicted above have laterally placed acrosomes. The presence of lateral acrosomes has distorted the appearance and shape of the sperm heads.

Number 1: Note that the acrosome of this sperm is situated laterally. As a result of this, the tapering sperm head has a distorted appearance. The midpiece is short but the tail is normal.

Number 2: The acrosome of this sperm is situated at the inferior and lateral position of the sperm head. As a result of this, the sperm head has the appearance of a bow pen. The midpiece is normal. The tail is normal.

AN UMBRELLA TYPE AND NORMAL ACROSOMES

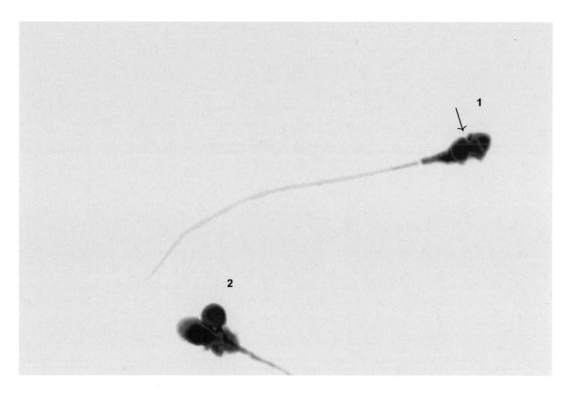

Figure 7.58: Rose Bengal and Toluidine blue stain (Oil immersion × 5000)

Number 1: These types of acrosomes are frequently associated with elongated sperm heads where the post-acrosomal portions of sperm nuclei exhibit a cone shaped elongation. Likewise, they are seen in a dumbbell shaped sperm heads. In this picture the conical acrosome covers the anterior portion of the sperm nucleus at the apex. The intact cytoplasmic margins are seen in the post-acrosomal portion of the nucleus (Arrow). The midpiece is thickened but the tail is normal.

Number 2: This picture illustrates a tapered sperm head. The post-acrosomal portion of the nucleus is asymmetrical. An irregular extrusion mass of cytoplasm, seen on either side of midpiece, is to be considered as normal. The acrosome, midpiece and tail are normal.

AN EARLY DETACHMENT OF ACROSOME

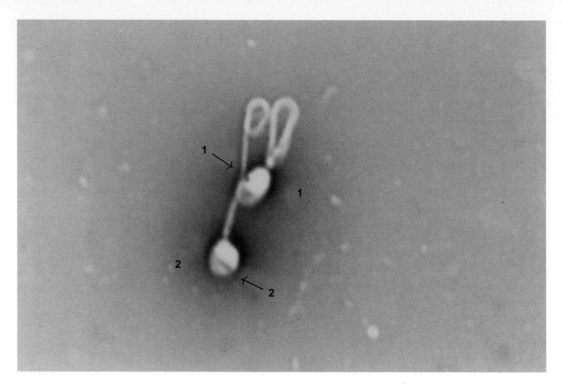

Figure 7.59: Eosin and Nigrosin stain (Oil immersion × 5000)

Number 1: A live sperm has a normal sperm head with a good distinction between the nucleus and the acrosome. At the upper margin of the post-acrosomal portion of the nucleus there is a notch, possibly indicating an invagination of cytoplasm into the nucleus (Arrow 1). The tail is coiled and rejoins itself at the midpiece region.

Number 2: This live sperm head shows an early detachment of the acrosome (Arrow 2). The sperm head, itself being non-oval, is abnormal. There is marked asymmetry of the post-acrosomal portion of the nucleus. There is eccentric attachment of the midpiece and the tail is curled at its terminal end.

A SEMI-DETACHED ACROSOME

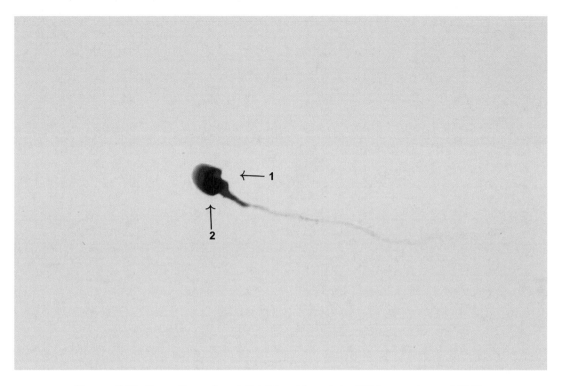

Figure 7.60: Rose Bengal and Toluidine blue stain (Oil immersion × 5000)

An acrosome is a double layered structure. This is seldom appreciated normally, in the stained preparations of semen. Rarely, the acrosome is partially detached from the nucleus as depicted above (Arrow 1). Then its double layered structure becomes apparent. In this case the thickened edge of the acrosome, along with its outer layer, is lifted up at the upper and right margin of the nucleus. This has exposed the inner layer of acrosome that is still attached to the nucleus. The half-lifted acrosome reveals the lower portion of the nucleus. The acrosome is still attached to the nucleus at its inferior margin (Arrow 2). The midpiece and tail are normal. The only other opportunity to appreciate the double layered structure of acrosome is available while studying the oversized acrosomes.

A SPERM WITH OVERSIZED ACROSOME

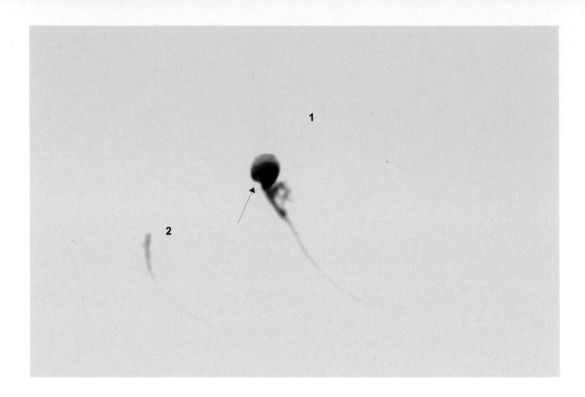

Figure 7.61: Rose Bengal and Toluidine blue stain (Oil immersion × 5000)

Number 1: This is a chance finding! It is infrequent but instructive aberration. It is, as if, the pyriform sperm head is wearing an oversized acrosomal helmet. There is a distinct gap between the left lateral margin of the nucleus and the acrosome (Arrow).

  Here is a unique opportunity for the investigator to perceive the double layered nature of acrosome consisting of the outer and inner layer. The midpiece is thick and shows a cytoplasmic extrusion mass, attached to it. The tail is normal.

Number 2: A pin headed sperm.

A PROTUBERANCE LIKE ACROSOME

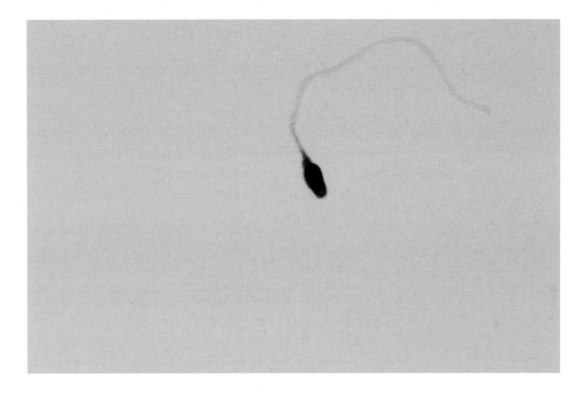

Figure 7.62: Rose Bengal and Toluidine blue stain (Oil immersion × 5000)

An elongated small sperm head shows a protuberance like acrosome at the apex. This type of acrosome is similar to, but not to be confused with, a "Nipple acrosome." The "Nipple acrosome" has a similar appearance and location but in addition it contains a central cyst. The acrosome depicted above does not have a central cyst. The midpiece is short but the tail is normal.

THE DIADEM DEFECT

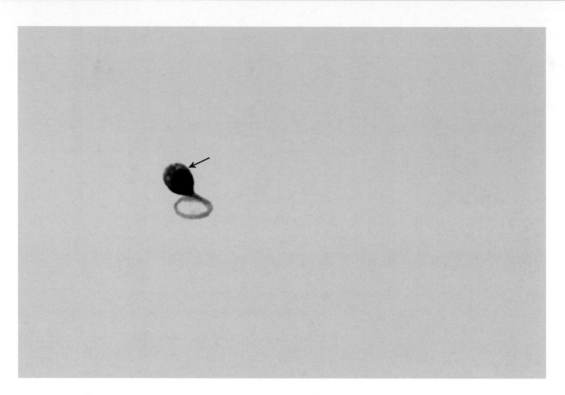

Figure 7.63: Rose Bengal and Toluidine blue stain (Oil immersion × 5000)

This picture illustrates the "Diadem Defect." The amorphous sperm head, with a short and coiled tail, shows a row of vacuoles around the sperm head positioned at the junction of acrocome and nucleus (Arrow). The name diadem is derived from the headband consisting of a circle of jewels worn by kings as a sign of sovereignty.

There are two types of vacuoles. The first type is produced by areas of defective condensation of the nuclear chromatin. The second type is produced by acrosomal invagination into the nucleus. The Diadem vacuoles are of the latter type. They are always membrane lined and have distinct boundaries.

A SPERM HEAD SHOWING DIADEM DEFECT

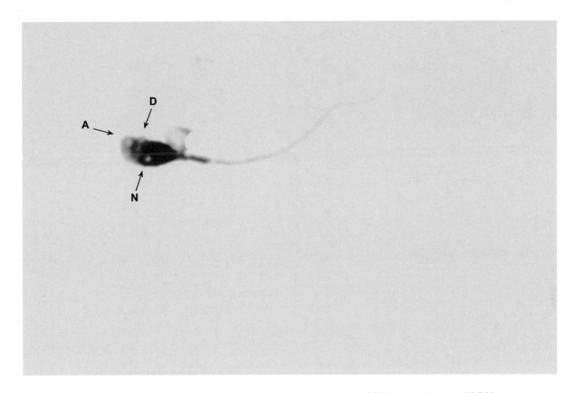

Figure 7.64: Rose Bengal and Toluidine blue stain (Oil immersion × 5000)

In this picture the sperm head, as if, is literally wearing a crown of vacuoles. The upper layer of vacuoles (Arrow A), shows the presence of two or three bigger sized acrosomal vacuoles. The lower layer of vacuoles (Arrow D) consisting of a row of four vacuoles, placed at the junction of acrosome and nucleus at the equatorial region, constitutes the "Diadem Defect."

The diadem means a headband of jewels worn by monarchs. The diadem vacuoles invariably are arranged in a row around the sperm head at the acrosome-nuclear junction.

The diadem vacuoles differ from the other nuclear vacuoles in that they are always membrane lined as they are produced by multiple invagination of acrosome into the nucleus. The membrane lining or the remnants of the same are seen only under an Electron microscope (Oettlé EE, Menkveld R and Swanson RJ et al., 1991).

A nuclear vacuole (Arrow N) is seen just below the equatorial region. Note the asymmetry of the post-acrosomal portion of the nucleus. The nuclear margins are slightly irregular. There is extrusion mass of cytoplasm attached to the midpiece that is otherwise normal. The tail is normal.

AN APICAL ACROSOMAL CYST

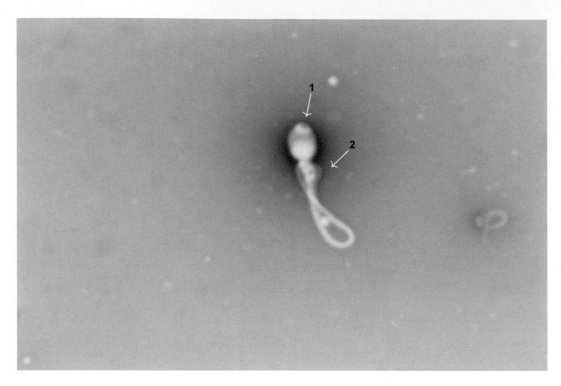

Figure 7.65: Eosin Y and Nigrosin stain (Oil immersion × 5000)

Oettlé EE, Menkveld R and Swanson RJ et al., (1991) have described in detail the morphology of an acrosomal cyst.

Eosin-Nigrosin viability stain offers a useful tool to visualize an acrosomal cyst. This picture shows an apical acrosomal cyst (Arrow 1). Note the lightly stained pink center is surrounded by a well-circumscribed white perimeter. The junction of the acrosome and the nucleus is clearly seen at the equatorial region.

The tail is curled upwards and ends in a loop with a cytoplasmic mass at the end. A small vacuole is seen in the midpiece region (Arrow 2).

AN ACROSOMAL CYST AND OTHER ABNORMALITIES

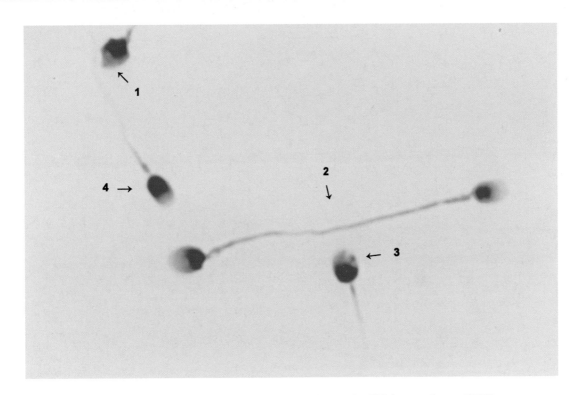

Figure 7.66: Rose Bengal and Toluidine blue stain (Oil immersion x 5000)

Number 1: This picture illustrates an amorphous sperm head with a triangular acrosome (Arrow 1). The post-acrosomal portion of the nuclear is irregular.

Number 2: This picture depicts a duplicate form resulting from end to end fusion of the two sperm tails (Arrow 2). Therefore, the net appearance of this form is that of a single tail with bipolar sperm heads.

Number 3: A sperm with normal oval sperm head shows the presence of an acrosomal cyst (Arrow 3). The cyst has a dark pink colored center surrounded by light pink colored perimeter. The cyst is produced by the acrosomal invagination into the nucleus. The junction line of the nucleus and the acrosome is seen below the cyst.

Number 4: This sperm has a small head with a normal acrosome but the midpiece and tail are normal.

LOCALIZED CONDENSATION OF ACROSOME

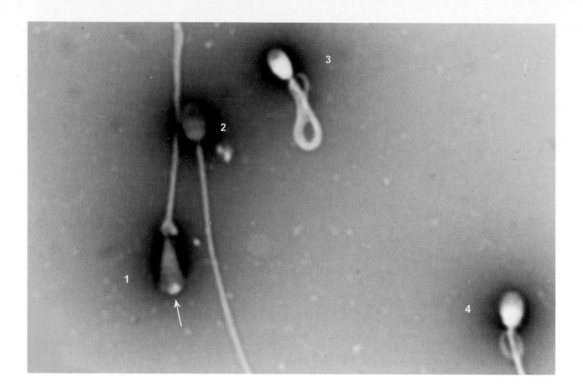

Figure 7.67: Eosin Y and Nigrosin stain (Oil immersion × 5000)

The Eosin-Nigrosin viability stain (Blom E 1950a), offers an excellent method for studying acrosomal abnormalities. The dead spermatozoa are stained pink while the living spermatozoa remain unstained white.

Number 1: The acrosome of this tapered sperm head shows a localized condensation at the apex (Arrow). The tail is thickened.

Number 2: This sperm has a normal oval head. However, the midpiece is thin and short. The tail is normal.

Number 3: A microsperm has a curled tail.

Number 4: This sperm has a normal oval sperm head with a normal acrosome. There is a mass of extruded cytoplasm encircling the midpiece but it is to be considered as normal.

A GIANT SPERM HEAD WITH MULTILOCULAR ACROSOME

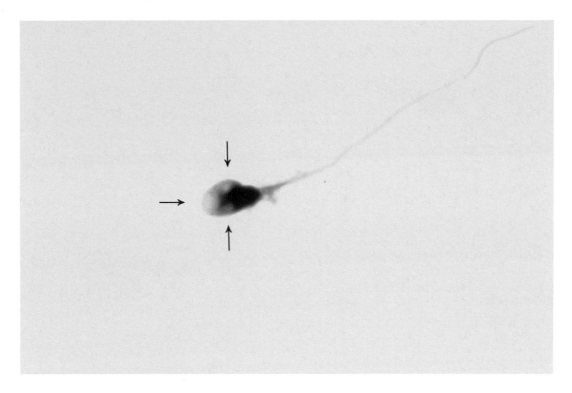

Figure 7.68: Rose Bengal and Toluidine blue stain (Oil immersion × 5000)

A giant sperm head of a megalosperm shows elongation of the post-acrosomal portion of the nucleus and a thickened neck. The acrosome covers the anterior half of the nucleus. It has a multilocular appearance due to the presence of three acrosomal cysts (Arrows). These cysts are well circumscribed. These pale stained cysts do not show evidence of acrosomal invagination. A small twig of cytoplasm is attached to the otherwise normal midpiece. Its tail is normal.

A MEGALOSPERM WITH RIDGED SPERM HEAD

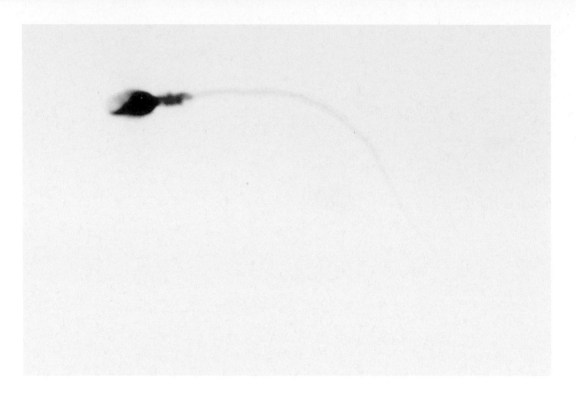

Figure 7.69: Rose Bengal and Toluidine blue stain (Oil immersion × 5000)

Oettlé EE, MenkveldR and Swanson RJ et al., (1991) have described the ridged sperm head in detail. It is due to the incomplete and abnormal separation of spermatids during spermiogenesis. Consequently the ridged sperm head is diploid or triploid. Usually, the two nuclei are either overlapping or are at right angles to each other. The extra nucleus appears as a central or lateral line running through the sperm head. The acrosome necessarily has a cleaved appearance. The nuclear material can be traced up to the tip. This picture depicts a ridged sperm head. In the original stained slide the two sperm nuclei, though not distinctly seen in this picture, were overlapping each other. The midpiece is thickened. The tail is normal.

A ROUND SPERM HEAD WITH CLEFT ACROSOME

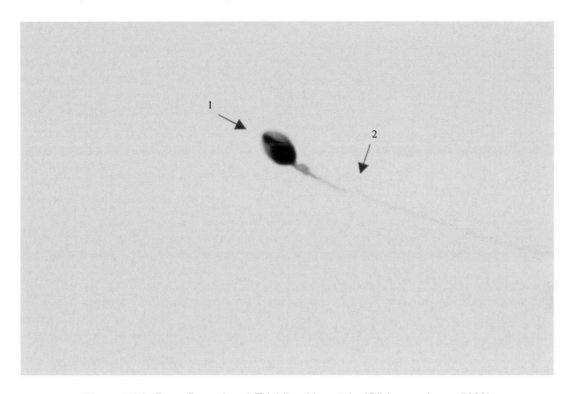

Figure 7.70: Rose Bengal and Toluidine blue stain (Oil immersion × 5000)

This sperm head is not to be confused with a ridged sperm head. The acrosome covering the nucleus is cleaved (Arrow 1). The upper margin of the round nucleus is easily discernible. A small twig of cytoplasm attached to the otherwise normal midpiece is not to be considered as an abnormality. The tail, slightly kinked at its junction with midpiece (Arrow 2), is otherwise normal.

DIFFERENT ACROSOMAL DEFECTS

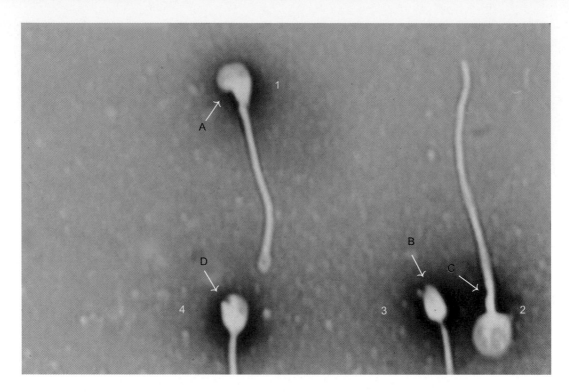

Figure 7.71: Eosin and Nigrosin stain (Oil immersion × 5000)

Number 1: This sperm head has a large acrosome that is tilted on one side (Arrow A). There is an abaxial attachment of midpiece to the head. The terminal end of the tail is looped.

Number 2: A large round sperm head has a large acrosome. The midpiece shows a notch at the side. (Arrow C) The tail is thick and short.

Number 3: A microsperm has a small acrososome (Arrow B). The midpiece is thin at the beginning but otherwise is normal.

Number 4: An acrosome of normal sperm head shows the presence of a notch (Arrow D). The neck joining the head and the midpiece is clearly seen.

PATCHY ACROSOME AND ACROSOMAL CYST

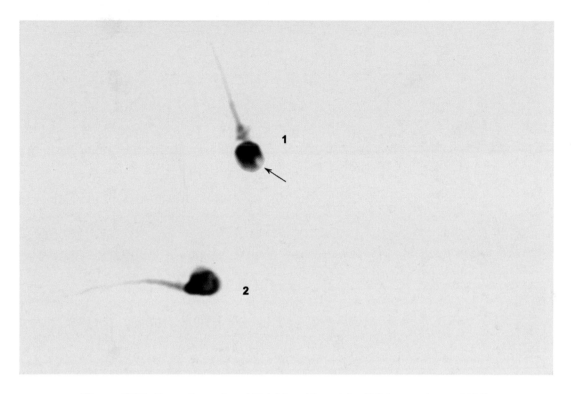

Figure 7.72: Rose Bengal and Toluidine blue stain (Oil immersion × 5000)

Number 1: An abnormal sperm has increased width of the post-acrosomal portion of the nucleus. The ratio of length to width exceeds 1.75. The acrosome shows a small apical cyst (Arrow). It has a lighter center and darker pink stained perimeter. The midpiece is attached slightly ab-axially but tail is normal.

Number 2: A pyriform sperm head has a patchy development of acrosome. The inner contour of the nucleus is visible through the acrosome. This could be a developmental defect as there is no other sign of degeneration of acrosome. The midpiece and tail are normal.

DISINTEGRATION OF ACROSOME

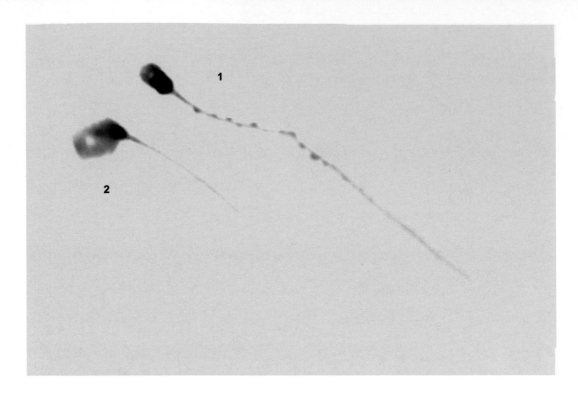

Figure 7.73: Rose Bengal and Toluidine blue stain (Oil immersion × 5000)

Number 1: An elongated sperm head has a normal acrosome. The midpiece is thin. The tail is long and has a beaded appearance.

Number 2: A disintegrating acrosome is depicted here. The acrosomal contents have escaped outside. The lower margin of the acrosome is faintly visible through the escaped acrosomal contents. The acrosomal matrix has probably escaped through a breach in the outer acrosomal layer leaving the inner acrosomal layer intact. This could be the beginning of the acrosomal reaction. The post-acrosomal portion of the nucleus appears to be normal. The midpiece and tail are normal.

AN ANOMALOUS DEVELOPMENT OF SPERMATID

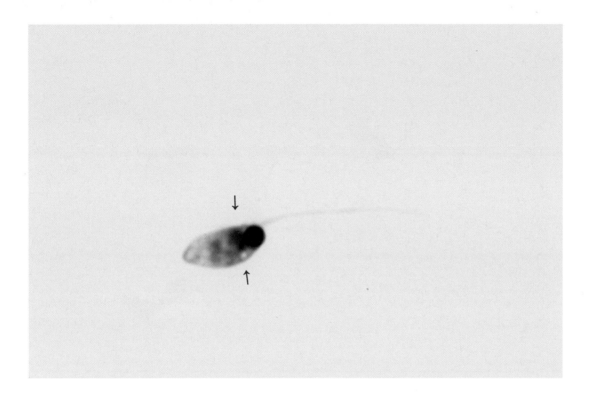

Figure 7.74: Rose Bengal and Toluidine blue stain (Oil immersion × 5000)

Logically this picture does not fit in the topic of "Acrosomal defects." In reality it depicts an anomalously developed spermatid that is likely to be confused for a sperm with a large acrosome. This is the only justification for its inclusion in the topic of acrosomal defects.

In this picture the central round nucleus of the elongated spermatid has migrated to one pole without undergoing concomitant nuclear changes characteristic of spermiogenesis. The acrosome has not developed. Just above the nucleus a pair of centrioles (Arrows'), at right angles to each other, and lying in the same plane, is seen. At the opposite pole a pseudo tail like process of cytoplasm is emerging out on the right. There is no neck or midpiece like structure. The nucleus is covered with a flame shaped mass of cytoplasm containing irregular pale vacuolated areas.

SPERM HEADS WITH THICKENED AND ELONGATED NECKS

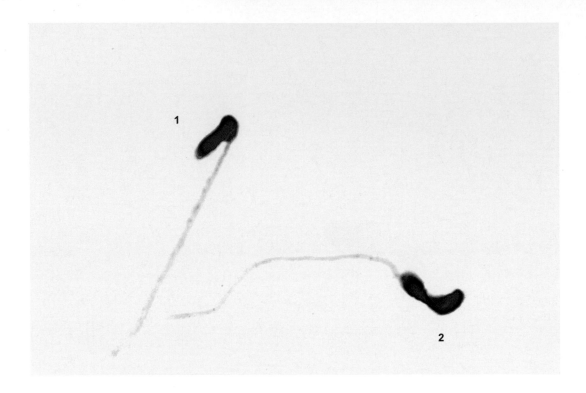

Figure 7.75: Rose Bengal and Toluidine blue stain (Oil immersion × 5000)

Number 1: This sperm has several defects. The elongated sperm head has a short acrosome and a thickened neck. Unlike WHO classification (1999) of sperm morphology, the Tygerberg classification has a separate subgroup of "Elongated heads" listed under sperm head defects. The midpiece is bent but still remains attached to the head. A small mass of residual cytoplasm is seen at the junction of the midpiece and sperm head. The tail is normal.

Number 2: This elongated sperm head has a normal acrosome, the post-acrosomal portion of the nucleus is elongated and the neck is elongated and bent. There is a residual mass of cytoplasm attached to the post-acrosomal portion of the nucleus and the terminal portion of the neck. The midpiece is bent. The tail is normal.

A SPERM WITH THICKENED NECK AND THIN MIDPIECE

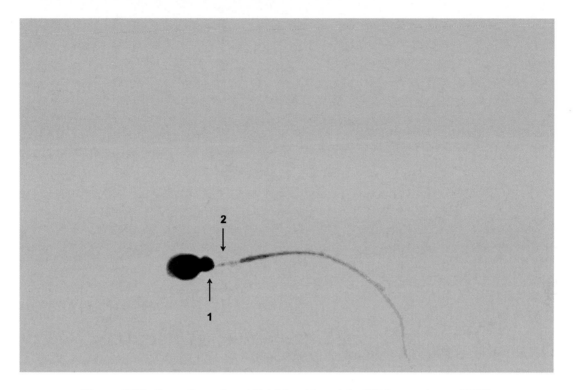

Figure 7.76: Rose Bengal and Toluidine blue stain (Oil immersion × 5000)

This picture of a sperm illustrates a non-oval sperm head with a normal acrosome and a thickened neck (Arrow 1).

The midpiece that is asymmetrically attached to the neck is thinner than the rest of the tail (Arrow 2). This type of lesion is seen due to a complete detachment of the mitochondrial sheath. Note that the detachment of mitochondria can be total or segmental.

SPERMS WITH BROKEN NECK AND BROKEN MIDPIECE

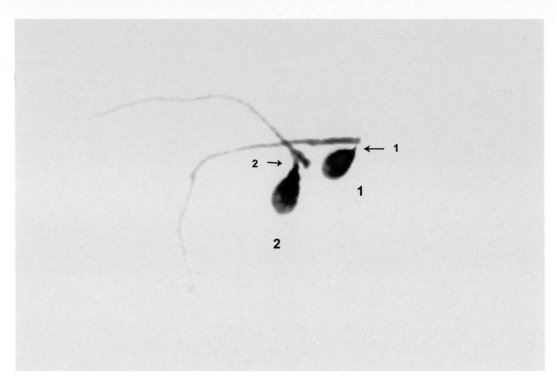

Figure 7.77: Rose Bengal and Toluidine blue stain (Oil immersion × 5000)

Number 1: A pyriform sperm head has a normal acrosome. The midpiece is broken. The acutely bent midpiece is detached from the sperm head (Arrow 1). This defect is due to a severe axonemal disruption including rupture and disorganization of fibrils (Acosta AA, Swanson RJ, Ackerman SB, Kruger TF, Menkweld R and van Zyl JA 1989).

Number 2: An elongated sperm head has a normal acrosome. The neck is broken. The separated midpiece is attached to the sperm head by means of a slender cytoplasmic stalk (Arrow 2).

Neither the WHO classification of sperm morphology (1999) nor the Tygerberg's classification of sperm morphology has taken cognizance of this defect.

A KINKED MIDPIECE AND A DETACHED MIDPIECE

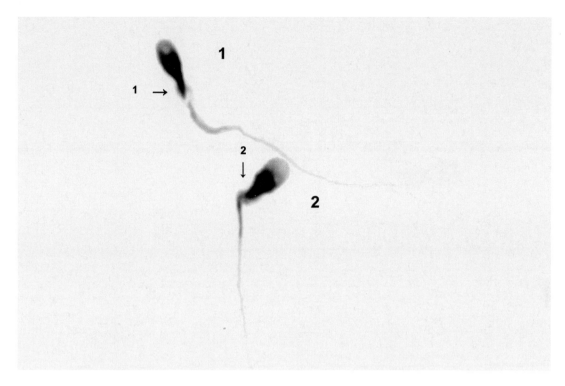

Figure 7.78: Rose Bengal and Toluidine blue stain (Oil immersion × 5000)

Number 1: Note that this elongated sperm head has a normal acrosome. There is a small twig of cytoplasm attached to the neck region. The curved and thickened midpiece is not attached to the sperm head (Arrow 1).

Number 2: This elongated sperm head has a normal acrosome. The midpiece, though centrally attached, is kinked and bent at a right angle (Arrow 2).

A SPERM WITH THICKENED AND IRREGULAR MIDPIECE

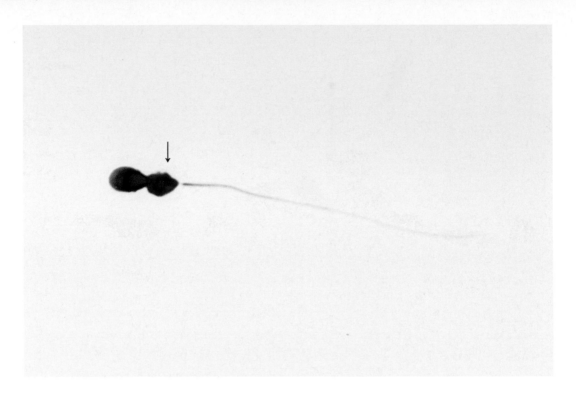

Figure 7.79: Rose Bengal and Toluidine blue stain (Oil immersion × 5000)

This pyriform sperm head measures 5.07 µm in length and 3.06 µm in width. The acrosome is normal. A mass of residual cytoplasm, greater than half the size of the sperm head, hence abnormal, is attached to the midpiece that is thickened and distorted (Arrow). The tail is normal.

There is little information available regarding the genesis of a "Pyriform" head. The author feels that a "Pyriform" sperm head is indicative of the nuclear immaturity. The rationale is as follows. The newly born spermatid has a central round nucleus. During spermiogenesis, the nucleus, first becomes "Pyriform" in shape corresponding to the Sb_2 stage (Heller and Clermont 1963), before undergoing elongation. Failure of this further nuclear development could naturally result in the "Pyriform" sperm head.

ASYMMETRICAL INSERTION OF MIDPIECE

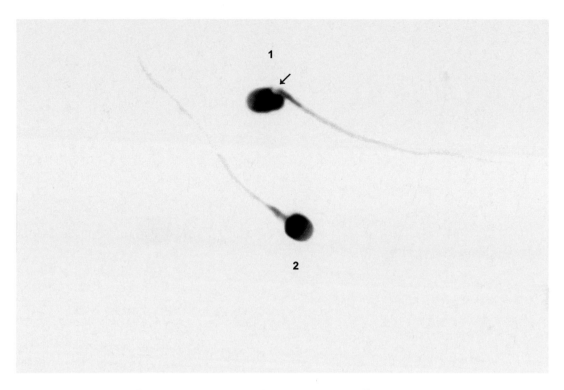

Figure 7.80: Rose Bengal and Toluidine blue stain (Oil immersion × 5000)

Number 1: This sperm head, with a thickened neck, has a small acrosome. The midpiece is implanted on the upper margin of the neck (Arrow). This is an extreme instance of asymmetrical attachment of the midpiece. The midpiece and tail are otherwise normal.

Number 2: This sperm has an amorphous non-oval sperm head with a normal acrosome. The midpiece and tail are centrally attached.

A SPERM WITH THICKENED MIDPIECE AND LONG TAIL

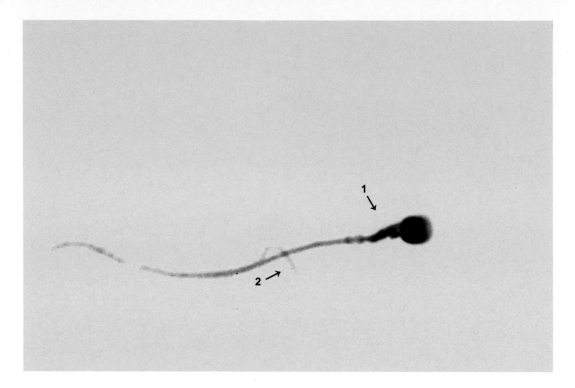

Figure 7.81: Rose Bengal and Toluidine blue stain (Oil immersion × 5000)

This sperm, with an amorphous head and a small acrosome, measures 4.05 μm in length and 3.35 μm in width. The ratio of length to width is 1.21. The thickened midpiece, (Arrow 1), has a length of 4.06 μm that is within normal limits. The width of the midpiece, which measures 1.41 μm, is increased (Normal 1 μm). The wavy thickened tail, measuring 41 μm in length, in reality is extra long, but because it is looped around itself, it appears to be normal. The terminal end of the tail (Arrow 2) is seen curving around the principal piece of the tail.

KINKED AND DETACHED MIDPIECES

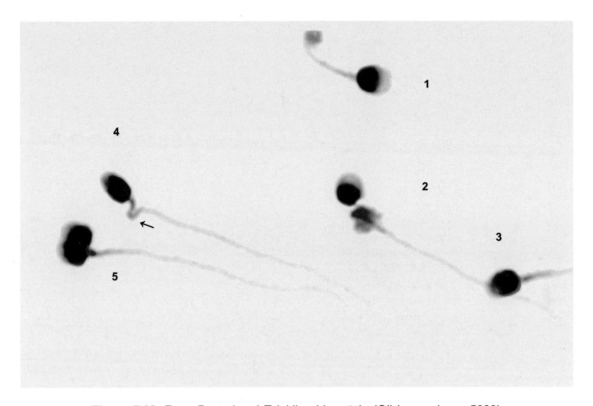

Figure 7.82: Rose Bengal and Toluidine blue stain (Oil immersion × 5000)

Number 1: A round headed sperm with normal midpiece and tail.

Number 2: A traumatic detachment of round head from the midpiece that is surrounded by irregular cytoplasmic extrusion mass. This could be an artifact. The tail is normal.

Number 3: An amorphous sperm head with altered length to a breadth ratio has a normal acrosome. The midpiece is normal.

Number 4: A microsperm with a small acrosome has a kinked midpiece (Arrow).

Number 5: This sperm has fused double heads with two separate acrosomes.

A GIANT HEAD WITH TWO CURLED TAILS

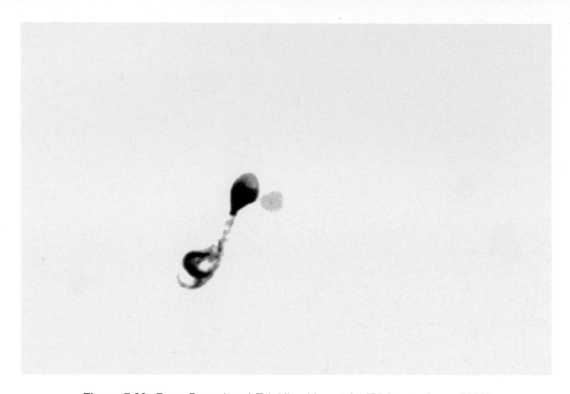

Figure 7.83: Rose Bengal and Toluidine blue stain (Oil immersion × 5000)

This sperm has multiple sperm abnormalities. The head is pyriform in shape. The post-acrosomal portion of the nucleus is asymmetrical. The neck is thickened. The middle piece is absent. Two short curled tails are directly attached to the neck. The terminal coiled portion of one tail is thickened. The tail margins (cell margins) are not continuous but are interrupted. A pink stained cytoplasmic droplet is seen near the sperm head.

AMORPHOUS SPERM HEADS WITH TAIL DEFECTS

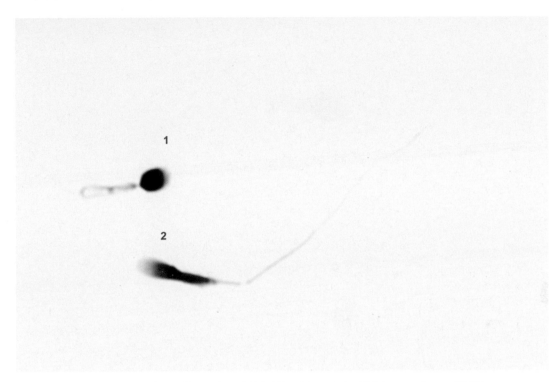

Figure 7.84: Rose Bengal and Toluidine blue stain (Oil immersion × 5000)

Number 1: A borderline sperm head is seen here. The length of the sperm head is 3.5 μm and its width is 2.6 μm. The ratio of the length to the width is 1.35. The tail is looped.

Number 2: This elongated sperm head has a length of 9.8 μm and its width is of 2.8 μm. The tail is bent at an angle lesser than < 90°.

Unlike WHO classification of sperm morphology (1999), Tygerberg classification has accorded a special identity to "Elongated sperm heads" under the "Sperm head defects" but has not given a subclassification.

Düsseldorf (1985, 1987 – refer Hoffman and Haider 1985, Hoffman et al., 1985, Hoffman 1987) has considered elongated spermatozoa as a result of a Sertoli cell dysfunction. As per his classification this sperm head would be included in "Type H-II°" wherein sperm heads exhibiting a cone shaped elongation of the post-acrosomal portion of the nucleus are to be included. According to him the "type HII°" defects are reversible.

SPERMATOZOA WITH DOUBLE TAILS AND DETACHED TAIL

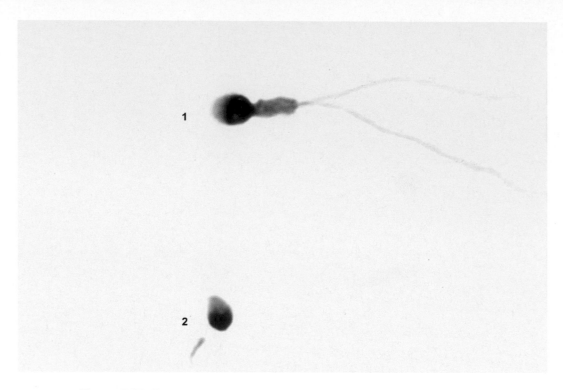

Figure 7.85: Rose Bengal and Toluidine blue stain (Oil immersion × 5000)

Number 1: A sperm with a large round head has a normal acrosome. The post-acrosomal portion of the nucleus is asymmetric. The neck is thickened. The midpiece is surrounded by a cytoplasmic residual mass and hence appears to be enlarged and irregular. The two tails are connected to the midpiece.

Number 2: A microsperm has an acrosome that is tapered anteriorly. There is no connection between the sperm head and the tail piece. This could be a result of an artifact produced during the preparation of the smear.

A SPERM WITH DOUBLE TAIL

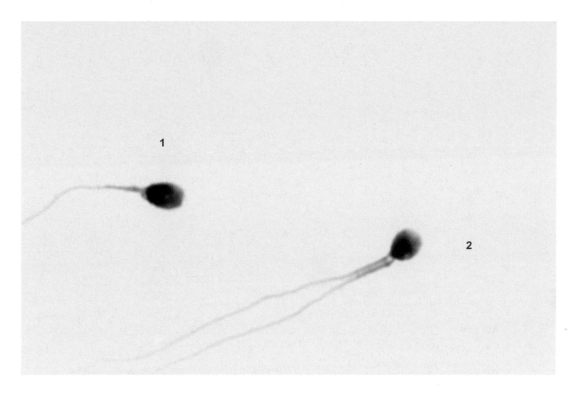

Figure 7.86: Rose Bengal and Toluidine blue stain (Oil immersion × 5000)

Number 1: This sperm has elongated head with a normal acrosome. The midpiece and tail are normal.

Number 2: This sperm has a pyriform head with a normal acrosome. The post-acrosomal portion of the nucleus is asymmetrical. Note the two separate midpieces and tails.

SPERMATOZOA WITH THICK TAILS

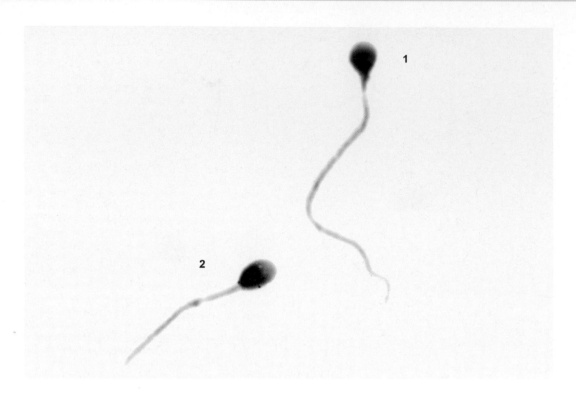

Figure 7.87: Rose Bengal and Toluidine blue stain (Oil immersion × 5000)

Number 1: This sperm that has a pyriform head, has a small acrosome. The midpiece is indistict in its lower part. The tail is thick in most of its principal part and is curled at the lower end.

Number 2: This sperm has an elongated head with normal acrososome. The midpiece is normal but the tail is thickened.

A SPERM WITH SEVERE "DAG" DEFECT OF THE TAIL

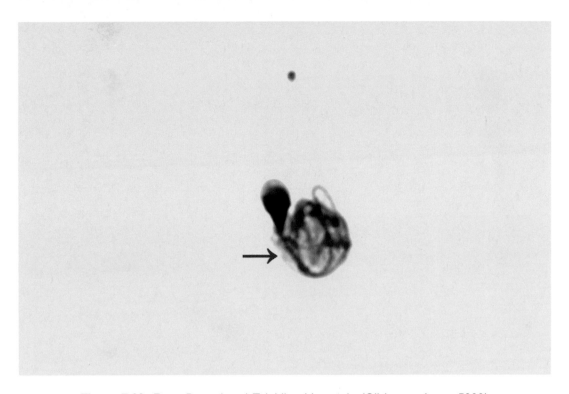

Figure 7.88: Rose Bengal and Toluidine blue stain (Oil immersion × 5000)

A sperm with an elongated head shows a severe "Dag" defect of the tail.

The "Dag" defect is not a common tail abnormality. The name 'Dag' is derived from a similar defect first described in a bull named Dag. This defect is characterized by coiling of the tail within an intact cytoplasmic membrane. Oettlè EE, Menkveld R, Swanson RJ et al., (1991).

This defect supposedly originates in the epididymis and not in the testis. There is rupture of fibrils and axonemal degeneration. Fibrils and mitochondria are lying loose in the enclosed cytoplasm.

In this picture the elongated sperm head has a normal acrosome. There is a cone shaped elongation of the post-acrosomal portion of the nucleus. A cytoplasmic spherical mass is seen in the midpiece region (Arrow). Multiple coils of the tail are seen in the cytoplasmic mass. The end piece of the tail is not visible.

THE "DAG DEFECT" OF TAIL

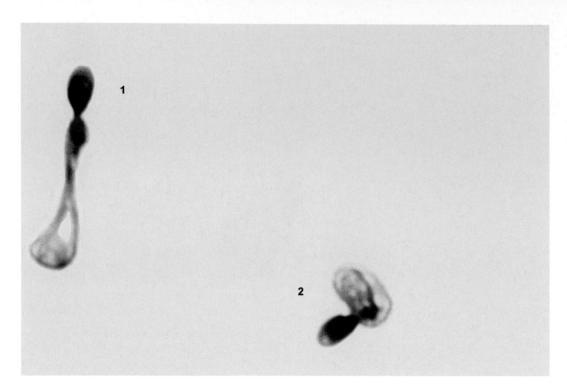

Figure 7.89: Rose Bengal and Toluidine blue stain (Oil immersion × 5000)

Number 1: A sperm having an elongated head with normal acrosome shows a severe "Dag defect" of the tail. The midpiece is masked by the tail ends. The two tails after coiling around a mass of cytoplasm are turned upwards and looped around the midpiece.

Number 2: This sperm has an elongated tapered head and a normal acrosome. The midpiece that is thickened and irregular shows three dark staining areas. The tail originating from the lowermost dark stained area curls around a vacuolated cytoplasmic mass.

MIDPIECE AND TAIL DEFECTS

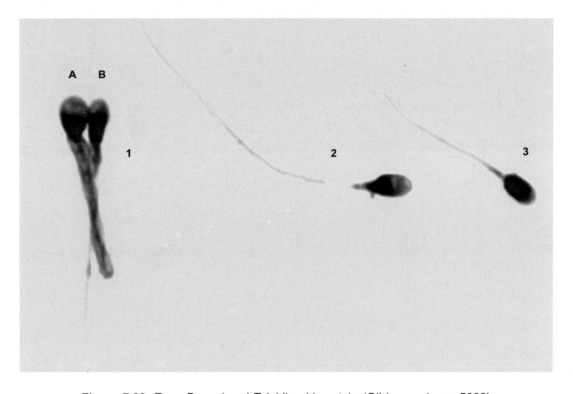

Figure 7.90: Rose Bengal and Toluidine blue stain (Oil immersion × 5000)

Number 1: An atypical duplicate form is illustrated here. Note that both the sperms are attached at the acrosomal and midpiece region. The individual sperm heads are dissimilar, one being pyriform (A) and the other being elongated (B). The midpieces are fused together. The sperm (A) has thickened midpiece and its tail shows hairpin as well as severe "Dag Defect." The tail that is coiled around and spirally twisted ends upward around the midpiece. The sperm (B) has thickened midpiece and its tail emerges out on a left side.

Number 2: An elongated spermatozoon with a normal acrosome shows a gap in the midpiece region. This broken midpiece could be an artifact.

Number 3: A sperm with elongated head has small acrosome but the midpiece and tail are normal.

SPERMATOZOA WITH RUDIMENTARY TAILS

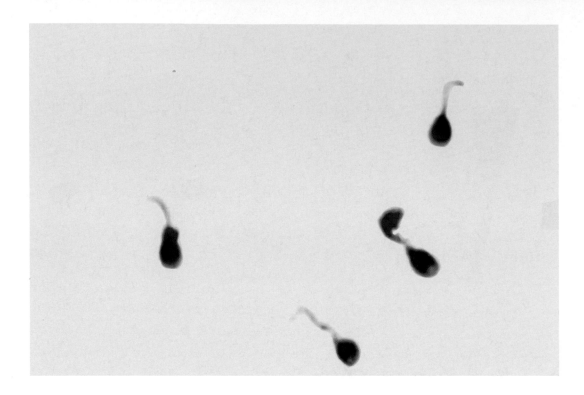

Figure 7.91: Rose Bengal and Toluidine blue stain (Oil immersion × 5000)

The picture depicts spermatozoa with rudimentary tails. Such types of tails are also called 'tadpole-like' tails. In Düsseldorf's classification (1985, 1987 – refer Hoffman and Haider 1985, Hoffman et al, 1985, Hoffman 1987) this type of defect is classified as Type III° defect. Needless to mention that such spermatozoa are non-motile.

SPERMS WITH NORMAL AND SHORT THICK TAILS

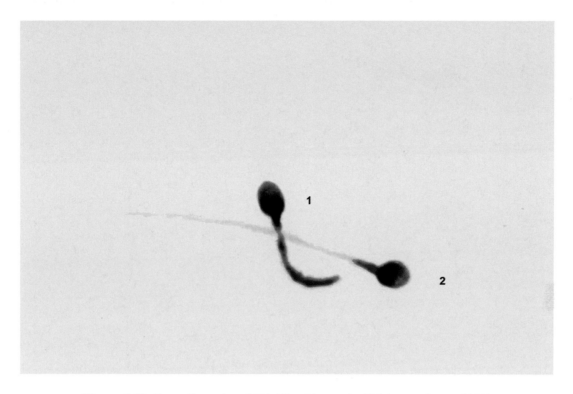

Figure 7.92: Rose Bengal and Toluidine blue stain (Oil immersion × 5000)

Number 1: This sperm has a normal oval head with a normal acrosome. The short midpiece is attached slightly ab-axially to the head. The curved tail is short and thick. Such sperms are non-motile.

Number 2: A sperm with a round head and normal acrosome has a normal midpiece and tail.

A SHORT TAIL AND A CURLED TAIL

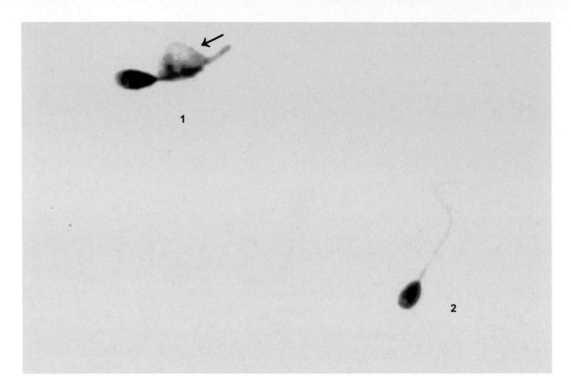

Figure 7.93: Rose Bengal and Toluidine blue stain (Oil immersion × 5000)

Number 1: This sperm has a tapered head that has a normal acrosome. The midpiece is thickened and a cytoplasmic remnant (Arrow) is attached to it. The size of the attached cytoplasmic remnant is bigger than that of the sperm head and hence it is to be considered as abnormal. The midpiece is thick and the tail is short.

Rarely one comes across a semen specimen of an infertile man wherein most of the sperms, if not all, manifest this type of abnormality. This could be a genetic defect and is incurable.

Number 2: A sperm with a small tapered head has a normal acrosome. Note the curling of the short tail at the endpiece region.

A DOUBLE TAIL WITH A HAIRPIN DEFECT

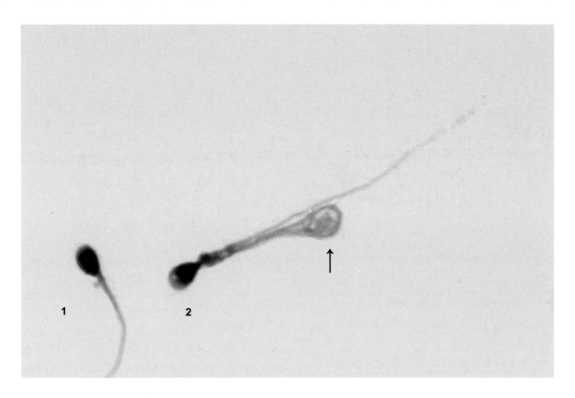

Figure 7.94: Rose Bengal and Toluidine blue stain (Oil immersion × 5000)

Number 1: A sperm with a small oval head and short acrosome has a normal midpiece and a thickened tail.

Number 2: Note that this sperm with pyriform head with normal acrosome has a short midpiece and two tails. The upper tail is normal. The lower tail (Arrow) shows a hairpin defect. The tail has coiled around a blob of cytoplasm and has turned upwards to its origin at the midpiece.

A CURVED MIDPIECE AND A BENT TAIL

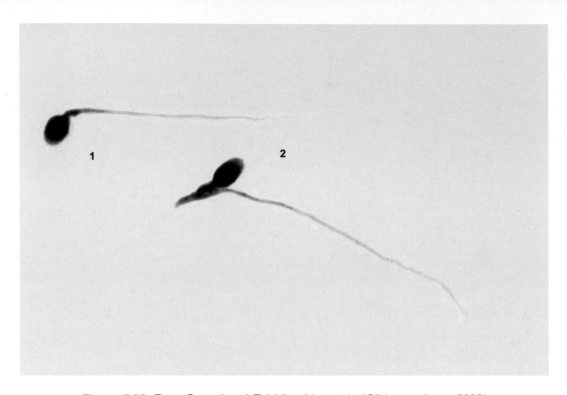

Figure 7.95: Rose Bengal and Toluidine blue stain (Oil immersion × 5000)

Number 1: This sperm has a small head with short acrosome. The midpiece is curved at its point of attachment to the head. The tail is normal.

Number 2: A sperm with a small elongated head has a short acrosome. The midpiece is normal but the tail is bent at an angle > 90°.

CURLED TAIL AND A HAIRPIN DEFECT OF TAIL

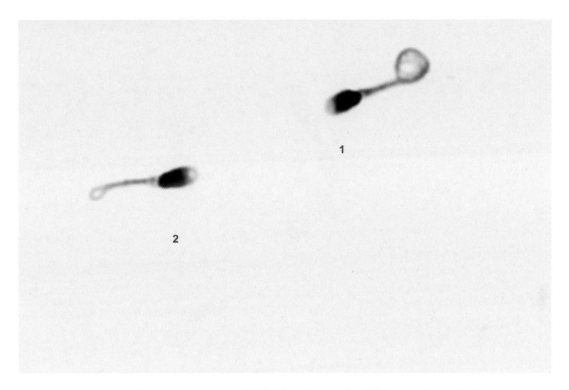

Figure 7.96: Rose Bengal and Toluidine blue stain (Oil immersion × 5000)

Number 1: An elongated sperm head with a normal acrosome has a curled tail.

Such curling of the tails is also seen in the hypo-osmotic swelling test (Jeyendran and Zeneveld 1986) that assesses the integrity of the cell membrane. When spermatozoa are exposed to hypo-osmotic conditions, fluid enters the spermatozoa in an attempt to maintain osmotic equilibrium. As a result of the fluid influx the sperm membranes swell. The tail fibrils that are already under tension, consequently curl up within the cell membrane. Such curling of tails can occur in any part of the tails. Such curled tails, seen as an end point of the hypo-osmotic swelling test, are similar in appearance to those depicted above. The curling of tails occurs due to transfer of fluid across the plasma membrane indicating the membrane integrity and normal function.

Number 2: This sperm shows a hairpin defect of the tail.

ROLLED TAILS, SHORT TAIL AND HAIRPIN LIKE TAIL

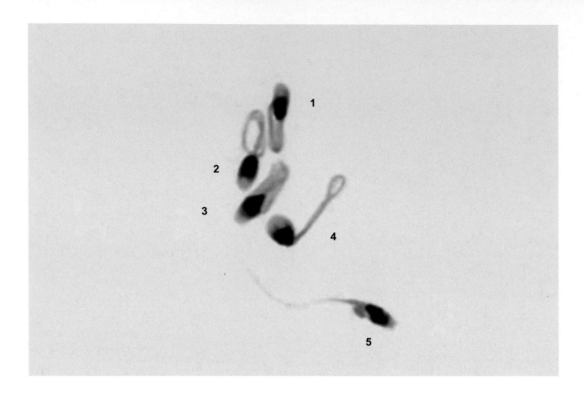

Figure 7.97: Rose Bengal and Toluidine blue stain (Oil immersion × 5000)

Numbers 1 and 2: These sperms have elongated heads with normal acrosomes. The midpieces are normal but the tails are rolled.

Number 3: This sperm has elongated head with normal acrosome. The midpiece is normal but the tail is coiled.

Number 4: A double headed sperm has a bent midpiece and its tail has a 'hairpin' like appearance.

Number 5: A sperm with abnormal head has a short acrosome. A residual remnant of cytoplasm is attached to the otherwise normal midpiece. The tail is short.

MULTIPLE TAIL ABNORMALITIES

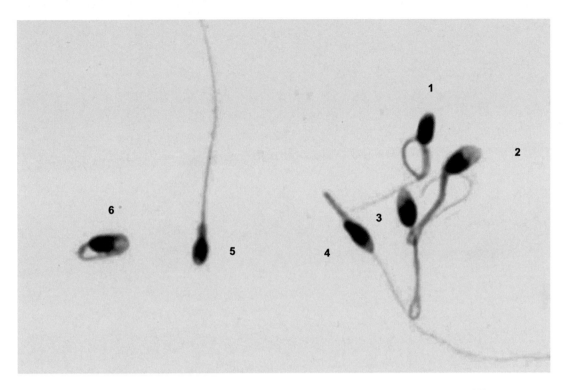

Figure 7.98: Rose Bengal and Toluidine blue stain (Oil immersion × 5000)

Number 1: A microsperm has a short acrosome. The tail is coiled.

Number 2: A double headed sperm with normal acrosomes has a thickened midpiece and a looped tail.

Number 3: A microsperm tapered anteriorly has a normal acrosome and shows a hairpin defect of the tail.

Number 4: This sperm, with an elongated head, has a normal acrosome. Its tail is bent at an angle > 90°.

Number 5: A microsperm has a normal midpiece and tail.

Number 6: The tail of this sperm, with elongated head and a normal acrosome, is and is seen going coiled around the head.

SPERMS WITH TAIL DEFECTS AND A SPERMATID

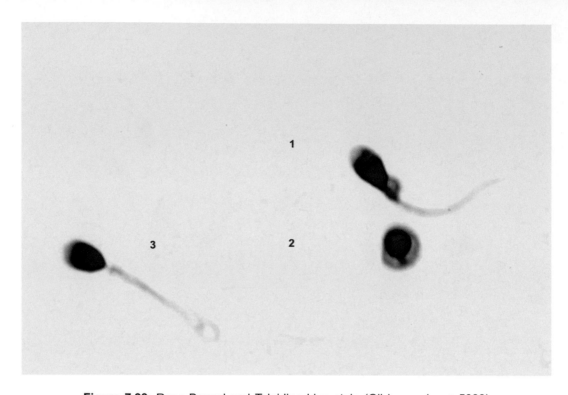

Figure 7.99: Rose Bengal and Toluidine blue stain (Oil immersion × 5000)

Number 1: A double headed sperm with a thickened midpiece has a short thick tail. A cytoplasmic twig is attached to the midpiece but it is to be considered as normal.

Number 2: A spermatid shows a normal acrosomal development.

Number 3: A large sperm head with a small acrosome shows a hairpin defect of the tail.

NORMAL, ABNORMAL SPERMS AND FREE HEADS

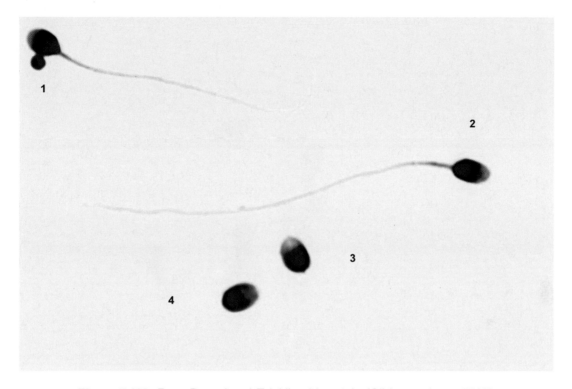

Figure 7.100: Rose Bengal and Toluidine blue stain (Oil immersion × 5000)

Number 1: This is a normal sperm.

Number 2: This sperm has an elongated head with a normal acrosome.

Numbers 3 and 4: Figures 3 and 4 illustrate the "Free" or "Loose heads." WHO Manual (Third edition 1990) had included such sperm heads under the neck and midpiece defects. However, in the fourth edition of WHO Manual (1999) such "Free heads" or "Loose heads" are not included under any of the Head, Neck, Midpiece or Tail defects.

In Tygerberg classification (1990), "Free heads" are included in secondary classification. Such heads are not considered as sperm abnormality but while recording are expressed as number of such "Free heads" per 100 spermatozoa counted.

CYTOPLASMIC REMNANTS ATTACHED TO THE MIDPIECE

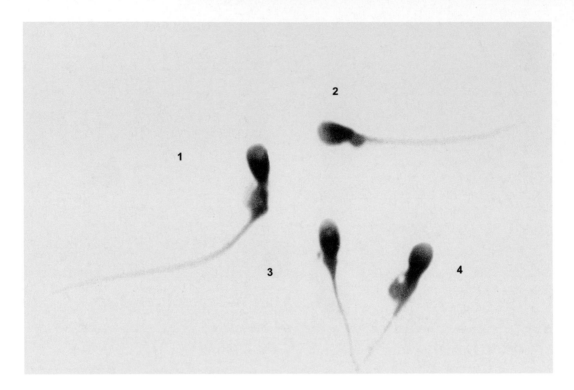

Figure 7.101: Rose Bengal and Toluidine blue stain (Oil immersion × 5000)

The common feature of all these sperms is the attachment of cytoplasmic remnants in the midpiece region.

When a spermatid is released from a Sertoli cell during spermiation, a cytoplasmic tag remains attached to it. This cytoplasmic tag is divided into two unequal parts. The smaller one, the cytoplasmic droplet, remains attached to the spermatozoon. The larger part, the residual body, is gradually separated. The cytoplasmic droplets have the same characteristics as that of the residual bodies.

According to WHO Classification (1999), the attached cytoplasmic remnants, if greater than one-third the area of the sperm head, are to be considered abnormal.

In this picture the cytoplasmic droplets, attached to the tapered form (No.2) and the microsperm (No.3), are to be ignored. The cytoplasmic remnants remaining attached to the midpiece regions of the sperms with an elongated (No. 1) and pyriform (No. 4) heads are indicative of sperm immaturity and point to epididymal pathology.

A CYTOPLASMIC MASS ATTACHED TO THE MIDPIECE

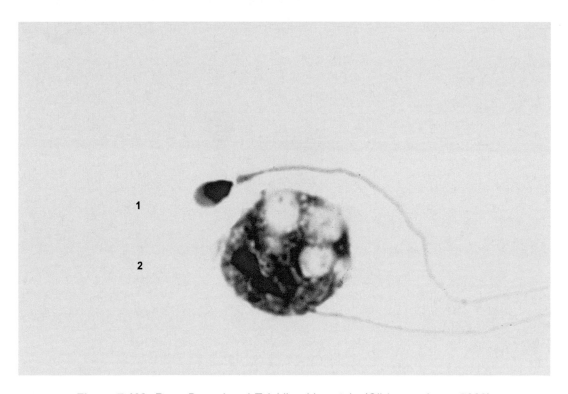

Figure 7.102: Rose Bengal and Toluidine blue stain (Oil immersion × 5000)

Number 1: A sperm with an elongated head shows a detached midpiece and a normal tail.

Number 2: A tapered sperm head with an elongated post-acrosomal portion of the nucleus shows a huge cytoplasmic mass attached to it in the midpiece region behind the nucleus. Note that the tapered sperm head, with indistinct acrosome, is not embedded in the cytoplasmic mass. The remnants of nuclear material are seen in attached cytoplasmic mass which shows fine and big vacuoles. The attached cytoplasmic mass has retained the pink stain.

IMMATURE SPERM CELL IN A CYTOPLASMIC MASS

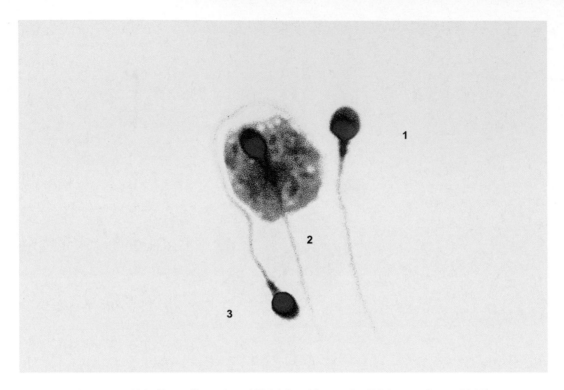

Figure 7.103: Rose Bengal and Toluidine blue stain (Oil immersion × 5000)

Number 1: This large head of the sperm shows asymmetry of the post-acrosomal portion of the nucleus. The acrosome, the midpiece and the tail are normal.

Number 2: This sperm has normal head with a small acrosome. The midpiece is thickened but the tail is normal. The entire sperm head, the midpiece and the proximal part of the tail are embedded in the cytoplasmic mass which shows few vacuoles.

Number 3: A normal sperm.

TAIL -TO- TAIL TYPE AGGLUTINATION OF SPERMS

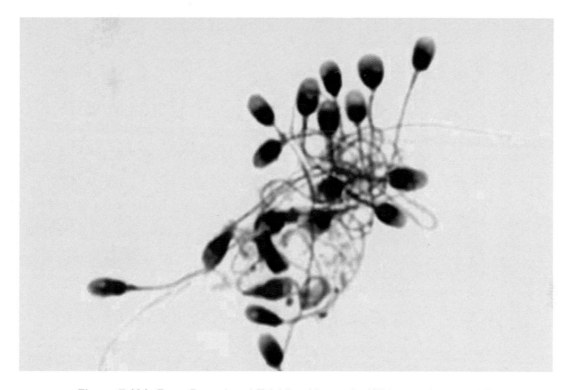

Figure 7.104: Rose Bengal and Toluidine blue stain (Oil immersion × 5000)

This picture illustrates a clump of sperms showing mainly the tail-to-tail type of agglutination of sperms in semen. The agglutination of sperms can be of three types, namely, of head-to-head type, mixed type and tail-to-tail type. Out of these tail-to-tail type of agglutination is important because it is indicative of the presence of sperm auto-antibodies in the blood sera of such patients.

Kibrick's method (Kibrick et al., 1952), also known as gelatin agglutination test, is universally used for detection of sperm autoantibodies in the sera of infertile men. It detects the presence of sperm agglutinins in the blood sera of the patients. In this test, the microscopic examination of the agglutinated clumps shows mainly tail-to-tail type of agglutination of sperms.

However, sperm agglutination also occurs due to the presence of bacteria, fungi or debris in the seminal plasma.

PIN HEADED SPERMATOZOA

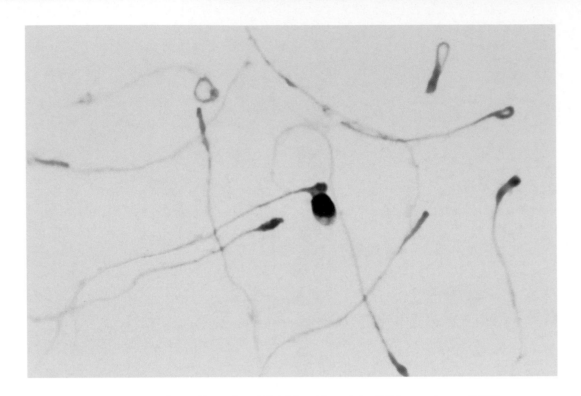

Figure 7.105: Rose Bengal and Toluidine blue stain (Oil immersion × 5000)

This picture illustrates spermatozoa with "Pin heads", excepting one normal form with bent midpiece at the center. The "Pin head" defect is an incurable one and is indicative of absolute sterility. Only the sperm morphology classification of Hotchkiss (1938) had a separate entity of "Pin heads" listed under sperm head defects.

WHO Manual (1999) states that the loose sperm heads lying free and "Pin heads" are not to be counted while assessing sperm morphology but are to be reported separately. The reason being that the "Pin heads" rarely possess a chromatin or a head structure and hence are not counted as sperm head defects.

As to the genesis of "Pin heads," the Manual states "Failure of the basal plate to attach to the nucleus at the pole opposite to acrosome causes the heads to detach on spermiation. The heads are absorbed and only the tails are found in semen giving "Pin head" defects." However, in "Pin heads" an intact basal plate is seldom seen. The WHO explanation is more applicable to the decapitated forms with intact basal plate, midpiece and single or multiple tails (See Figure 7.30).

Interestingly, Mann (1964) had reported "Pin head" spermatozoa in a case of sterile Guernsey bull.

A BINUCLEATE SPERMATID WITH A TAIL

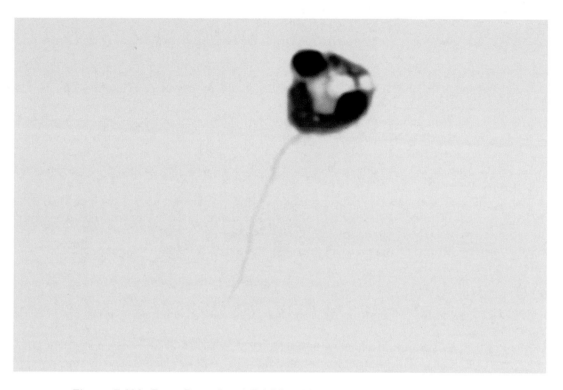

Figure 7.106: Rose Bengal and Toluidine blue stain (Oil immersion × 5000)

This picture illustrates a binucleate spermatid with a tail. Note that the cytoplasm of the spermatid contains three to four vacuoles. At the lower margin remnants of cytoplasmic reticulum are seen (Arrow). The upper nucleus is not round but has assumed a "sperm head" like shape. It is devoid of acrosome.

The lower nucleus has an oval appearance akin to a sperm head but is devoid of any acrosome. From the lower end of this nucleus the tail is emerging out.

BIBLIOGRAPHY

1. Acosta AA, Swanson RJ, Ackerman SB, Kruger TF, Menkweld R, van Zyl JA. (Eds): Human Spermatozoa in Assisted Reproduction. Williams and Wilkins. Baltimore 1989.
2. Baccetti B, Renieri T, Rosati F, Selmi MG, Casanova S. Further observations on morphogenesis of round headed spermatozoa. Andrologia 1977;9:255.
3. Bartoov B, Elites F, Langsman J, Synder M, Fosher J. Ultrastructure studies in morphological assessment of human spermatozoa. Int J Androl Suppl 1982;5:81.
4. Blom E A one minute live dead sperm stain by means of Eosin-Nigrosin. Fertil Steril 1950a; 1: 176.
5. David G, Bisson JP, Jouannet PC, et al. Les teratospermies. In Thiboult C (Ed): La sterilitie due male. Aquisions recents. Masson et cie Paris 1972.
6. Fredricson B, Bjork R. Morphology of post-coital spermatozoa in the cervical secretions and its clinical significance. Fertil Steril 1977;28:841.
7. Heller CG, Clermont Y. Spermatogenesis in man: an estimate of its duration. Science 1963;140:184.

8. Hofmann N, Freundl G, Florack M. Die Formsörungen der Spermatozoen im Sperma und Zervikalschleim als spiegel testicuärer Erkankungen, Gyäkologe 1985;18:189.

9. Hofmann N, Haider SG. Naue Ergebnisse morphologischer Diagnosticks der Spermatogenestörungen. Gynaäkologe 1985;18:70.

10. Hofmann N. Wege Zur Andrologie, Winführung in die Praxis, Erester Teil. Bremenhaven : Ditzen Druck und Verlgas- G M BH 1987.

11. Holstein AF, Schirren C, Schirren CG. Human spermatids and spermatozoa lacking acrosomes. J Reprod Fertil 1973;35:489.

12. Jaunnet P, Ducot B, Feneux D, Spira A. Male factor and the liklihood of pregnancy in infertile couples.1, Study of sperm characteristics. Int J Androl 1988;11:379.

13. Jayendra RS, Zenevel LJD. Human sperm hypo-osmotic test.Fertil Steril 1986;46:151.

14. Kibrick S, Belding DL, Merril B. Methods for detection of autoantibodies against mammalian spermatozoa: gelatib agglutunation test. Fert Steril 1952;3:430.

15. Liu DY, Baker HWG. Morphology of spermatozoa bound to the zona pellucida of human oocytes that failed to fertilize in vitro. J Reprod Fertil 1992;94:71.

16. Macleod J. The significance of deviation in human sperm morphology in human testis. Adv. Exp. Med. Biol 1970;10:481.

17. Mann T. Spermatozoa :Structural and Functional Characteristics; Motility and Fertility. In: The Biochemistry of semen and of the male reproductive tract. Metuen and company. London 1964;p.22.

18. Menkveld R, Franken DR, Kruger TF, Oehninger S. Sperm selection capacity of the human zona pellucida. Mol. Reprod. Dev 1991;30:346.

19. Meschede D, Keck C, Zander M, Cooper TG, Young CH, Vieschlag E. Influence of three different preparation techniques on the results of human sperm morphology analysis. Int. J. Androl 1993;16:33.

20. Mortimer D, Leslie EE, Kelley RW, Templeton AA. Morphological selection of human spermatozoa in vivo and in vitro. J. Reprod. Fertil 1982;64:391.

21. Oettlé EE, Menkveld R, Swanson RJ, Oehninger S, Fruger TF, Acosta AA. Photomicrographs with interpretation. In : Menkveld R, Oettlè EE, Kruger TF, Swanson RJ, Oehninger S (Eds): Atlas of Human Sperm Morphology. Williams and Wilkins. Baltimore. Diadem defect 1991; p. 27,62, 86. Acrosomal cyst p.76. Dag defect pp. 45, 48, 54.

22. Phadke AM. Supravital staining technique for semen. Andrologia 1978;10:80.

23. World Health Organization. WHO Laboratory manual for the examination of human semen and sperm-cervical mucus interaction. 4th edn. Cambrdge University Press. Cambridge 1999.

24. Zaneveld LJD, Polakashi. Collection and physical examination of the ejaculate. In Hafez ESE (Ed): Techniques of Human Andrology. Elsevier/North Holland, Amsterdam. 1977;p.147.

Pyospermia

Meaning and definition of pyospermia.
The role of infection in male infertility.
Significance of pyospermia.
Methods used for the evaluation of pyospermia.
Activation of WBCs in the male genitourinary tract.
The constituent cells and their origin in pyospermia.
Confusion between the inflammatory cells and the immature germ cells.

PYOSPERMIA

MEANING AND DEFINITION OF PYOSPERMIA

The term "Pyospermia" is used when significant number of leukocytes are present in the semen. "Leukospermia" and "Pysemia" are other terms synonymously used.

WHO Manual (1999) states that the concentrations of WBCs greater than 1×10^6/cc are considered as elevated and the ejaculate is termed "Leukocytospermic."

The occurrence of 1-3 leukocytes per HPF in the semen is a normal finding. As a rough guide the presence of 5-10 or more of the leukocytes per HPF in the semen signifies pyospermia.

THE ROLE OF INFECTION IN MALE INFERTILITY

The infections of the male genital tract can be a causative factor in male infertility (Eliasson 1977; Fowler 1981)

White blood cells are deleterious because of their ability to stimulate reactive oxygen species (ROS), thereby reducing the sperm motility and function. Infections of epididymis (either gonococcal, filarial and/ or due to smallpox and tuberculosis) often lead to obstructive azoospermia. Infections of the prostate characterized by slightly reduced volume and low zinc content of the ejaculate, can lead to severe oligozoospermia or even azoospermia. Infection of seminal vesicles (Commonly tubercular) results in a substantial reduction of the volume and fructose content of the ejaculate.

SIGNIFICANCE OF PYOSPERMIA

Is Pyospernia Specific of Male Genital Tract Infections?

The presence of large number of leukocytes in semen though suggestive, is not specific of infection. Many men with WBC concentrations greater than 1×10^6/ml in gemen have normal semen variables. Studies have not shown association between bacteria growing in reproductive tract fluids, like semen, urine, and expressed prostatic secretions, and pyospermia (Jarvi and Noss 1994). Even chlomiphene citrate therapy can result in non-bacterial pyospermia (Matthews et al., 1995). Pyospermia is also observed in the initial semen samples following successful surgical procedures like Vaso-epididymostomy and recanalization of an obstructed vas deferens (Phadke AM 1975).

Appropriate Culture Tests are Necessary

Since pyospermia is potentially indicative of male genital infections, appropriate culture tests are indicated. Apart from sexually transmitted diseases (STD or venereal diseases) common infections include *Streptococcus fecalis, E. coli, Mycobacterium tuberculosis*, Chlamydia and Ureaplasma infections. Clinically silent prostatitis and epididymitis may exist in men without overt symptoms. In such conditions a bacterial origin must be suspected.

A semen culture and a urethral swab culture are used for suspected Chlamydia, Ureaplasma and Mycoplasma infections. Chlamydia infections in males cause epididymitis and are likely to be transmitted to the female partners who in turn may suffer from salphingitis.

Viruses that can be isolated from human semen include HIV I and II, Hepatitis B, Cytomegalovirus (CMV) and A Human papillomavirus (HPV).

METHODS USED FOR THE EVALUATION OF PYOSPERMIA

Papanicolaou Stain

In the Papanicolaou stained semen smear, the cytoplasm of leukocytes and macrophages is stained basophilic (green) while the cytoplasm of germinal cells is stained acidophilic (pink). The cytoplasm of the epithelial cells is variably stained.

Peroxidase Test

Proxidase tests performed on wet mounts of fresh semen are inexpensive and highly reliable. This test detects the peroxidase enzyme present in the polymorphonuclear leukocytes but does not detect other white blood cells in semen.

Immunohistocytology using Monoclonal Antibodies

Immunohistocytology enables quantitation of total white blood cells in semen and their individual subtypes by detecting WBC phenotype antigen with specific monoclonal antibodies (Eiserman et al., 1989; El-Demiry et al., 1986). This is relatively time consuming and expensive test.

Granulocyte Elastase and Cytokine Enzyme Linked Immunoabsorbant Assays

Granulocyte elastase is an enzyme specific to PMN leukocytes. This assay is quantitative and suitable for testing frozen semen specimens.

A number of pro-inflammatory cytokines have been detected in the seminal plasma. There is a positive association between leukocytospermia and elevated levels of interlukin-1B (Anderson DJ, 1997).

Chemiluminescence Assays

This assay is recently introduced for the detection of GUI (Kovalaski N. et al., 1991; Leino L and Virkkumen P. 1991; Krausz C et al., 1992). It detects super oxide radical formation after generation of ROC by activated PMN leukocytes. However, it is very expensive and not useful in clinical practice.

ACTIVATION OF WHITE BLOOD CELLS IN THE MALE GENITOURINARY TRACT

The white blood cells in the male genitourinary tract become activated by trauma, sperm antigens, products of microorganisms and viruses.

CONSTITUENT CELLS AND THEIR ORIGIN IN PYOSPERMIA

Though PMN leukocytes are dominant in pyospermia, other cells like microphages, macrophages (Mononuclear and multinucleate), tissue histiocytes and T lymphocytes also participate in the inflammatory response. In response to traumatic injury and in acute infections - both bacterial and viral- PMN leukocytes are the dominant cell type. In chronic infections and in response to sperm antigens, the presence of fair number of macrophages and T lymphocytes are observed in the inflammatory exudate. The role of macrophages in the cell mediated immunity is well known.

In the absence of urethritis, most of the inflammatory cells originate from epididymis, prostate and seminal vesicles.

CONFUSION BETWEEN THE INFLAMMATORY CELLS AND THE IMMATURE GERM CELLS

Confusion between these two types of cells is proverbial and notoriously common. Multinucleate spermatids are confused with polymonuclear leukocytes. Similarly spermatocytes are mistaken for lymphocytes and mono- and multinucleate macrophages. Unnecessary antibiotic therapy is given when immature germ cells are mistaken as the so called "pus cells."

In a case of obstructive azoospermia, if the presence of pus cells in semen is erroneously diagnosed as the presence of immature germ cells, a mistaken diagnosis of a non-obstructive azoospermia is reached and the patient is denied an opportunity of undergoing surgery for the removal of obstruction.

In clinical practice, a properly stained seminal smear either with Papanicolaou stain or modified Shorr stain will clear the oft-repeated mistake of labeling the immature germ cells as pus cells.

The next few pictures will illustrate this point.

PUS CELLS IN SEMEN

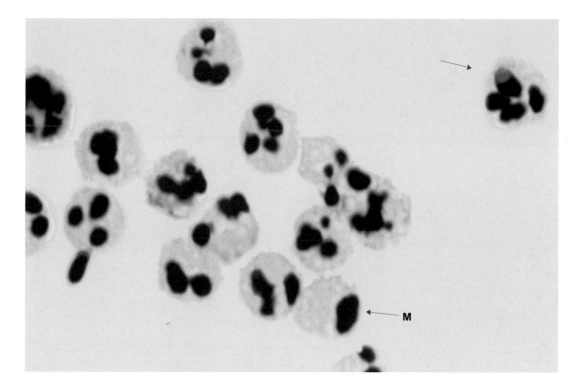

Figure 8.1: Papanicolaou stain (Oil immersion × 5000)

The term pyospermia indicates the presence of large number of leukocytes in the semen and is indicative of genital tract infection. Inflammatory lesions of testes, epididymis, seminal vesicles, prostate and urethra can lead to pyospermia.

The inflammatory cells though mainly consist of polymorphonuclear leukocytes, also include lymphocytes, plasma cells, monocytes, large and small macrophages and tissue histiocytes. The simultaneous presence of red blood cells and bacteria is uncommon in pyospermia.

Note that the interconnecting bands of multilobed nuclei of polymorphs may not be always seen. With Papanicpolaou stain the cell cytoplasm is stained bluish green and the nuclei are stained blue. The presence of the ingested sperm head (Arrow) in the cytoplasm of polymorphonuclear leukocytes, though very uncommon, is not unusual.

A mononuclear macrophage cell is also seen (Arrow M).

LEUKOCYTES WITH INGESTED SPERM HEAD

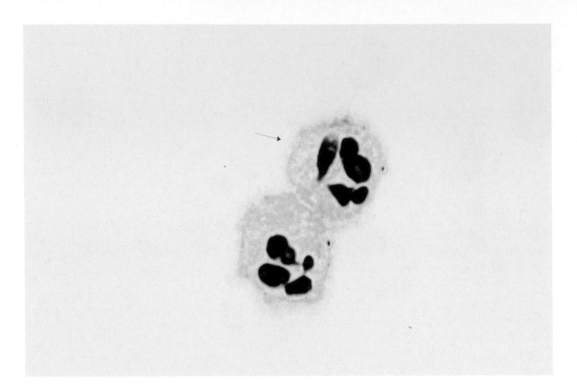

Figure 8.2: Papanicolaou stain (Oil immersion × 5000)

An exodus of the polymorphonuclear leukocytes from the tissue capillaries to the site of infection is the body's chief mechanism in combating infection. This constitutes body's first line of defense. Polymorphonuclear leukocytes are known to phagocytose the bacteria, cellular debris etc.

However, one often sees polymorphonuclear leukocytes with ingested sperm heads. In the Papanocolaou stained preparation the cytoplasm is stained green or bluish green. The nuclei are stained blue. The granules in the cytoplasm are clearly seen. In this picture an ingested sperm head in the cytoplasm of a polymorphonuclear leukocyte is clearly seen. WBCs are known to be activated by sperm antigens in the male genitourinary tract.

Gopalkrishnan et al., (1989) by Transmission Electron Microscopy studies of semen in genital tract infection, have demonstrated phagocytosed sperm head in a digestive vacuole of Neutrophils.

SUPRAVITAL STAINING OF PUS CELLS

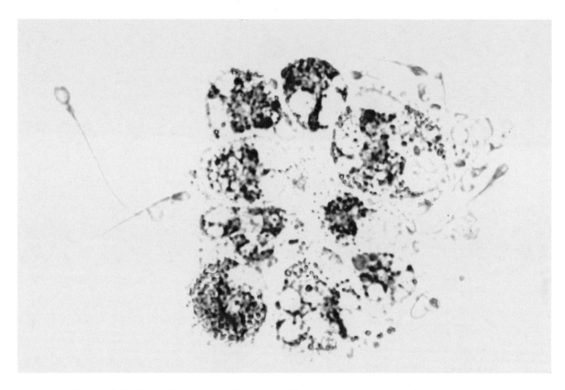

Figure 8.3: Neutral red supravital stain (High power 40x. Magnification × 2000)

This picture illustrates pus cells stained supravitally (Phadke 1978). Spermiophage cells and pus cells have the unique ability of absorbing the Neutral red dye in a weak solution and concentrating and storing it in their cell cytoplasm in the form of granules or globules.

Note that the supravital staining involves the staining of the cells in the living condition. The cell nuclei remain unstained. Staining of the nuclei indicates the death of the cell. Note that in the above picture the nuclei of polymorphonuclear leukocytes have remained unstained. Pink stained neutral red granules are visible in the cell cytoplasm of these cells. Spermatids in the semen remain unstained. Less experienced technicians, more often than not, confuse the spermatids for pus cells and consequently unnecessary antibiotic treatment is instituted. Reversely, in cases of obstructive azoospermia the presence of pus cells in semen is often being mistakenly reported as the presence of spermatids rendering a false diagnosis of non-obstructive azoospermia.

A MACROPHAGE CELL WITH INGESTED BACTERIA

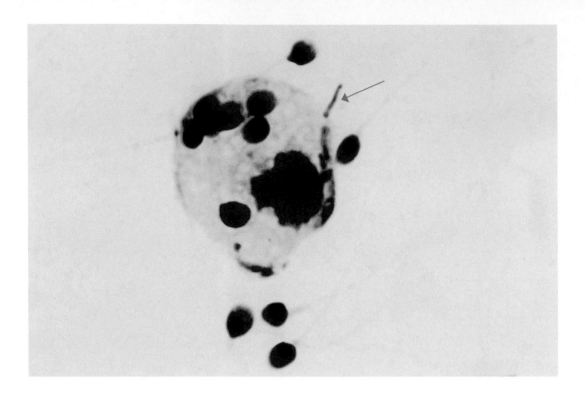

Figure 8.4: Papanicollaou stain (Magnification × 5000)

A macrophage cell with a diameter of 22.2 microns has a knob shaped nucleus at one end. The cytoplasm shows fine and coarse vacuoles and shows ingested sperm heads on the left. Inside the right margin of the cell, ingested bacilli are seen (Arrow). The tails of spermatozoa are indistinct.

A MONONUCLEAR MICROPHAGE CELL

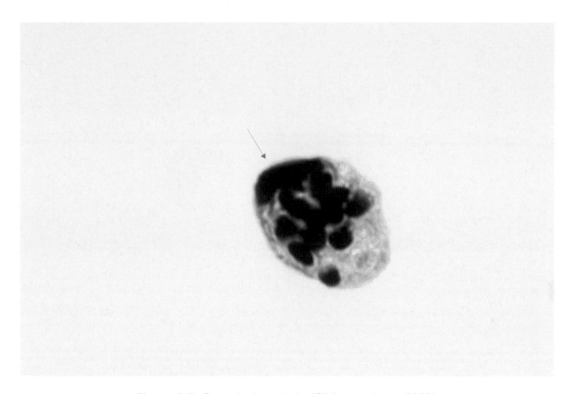

Figure 8.5: Papanicolaou stain (Oil immersion × 5000)

A mononuclear microphage cell measuring 19.4 microns × 15.4 microns has a crescent-shaped eccentric nucleus at the top (An arrow). The cell margins are regular. The cytoplasm that is stained green shows few vacuoles near the upper right border and numerous ingested sperm heads.

A MONONUCLEAR HISTIOCYTE

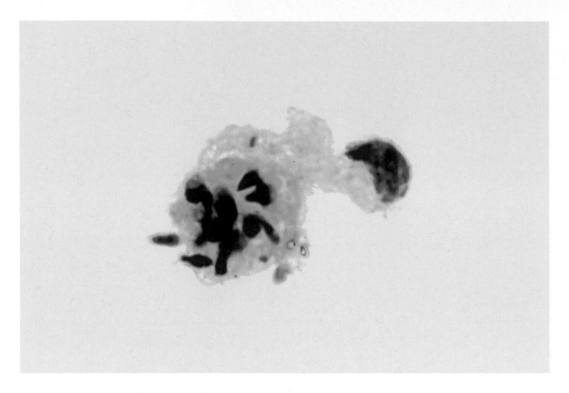

Figure 8.6: Modified Shorr stain (Oil immersion × 5000)

A mononuclear histiocyte has an eccentric sickle shaped nucleus at the extreme end on the right. The cell margins are irregular. The cytoplasm that is stained bluish green shows the a clump of ingested sperms on the left. Few tails are seen emerging out. Note the finely vacuolated cytoplasm.

A BINUCLEATE VACUOLATED MACROPHAGE CELL

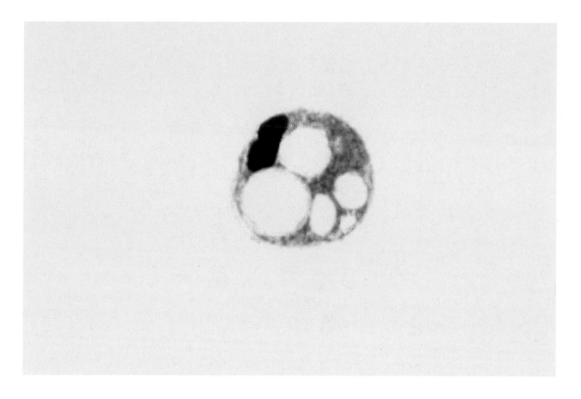

Figure 8.7: Papanicolaou stain (Oil immersion × 5000)

The cytoplasm of a binucleate round macrophage cell is stained intense green. The cell margins are regular. At eleven o'clock position the two nuclei, adjacent to each other, are situated. Five big vacuoles, in addition to the few fine vacuoles, are seen in the cytoplasm.

A GIANT BUNUCLEATE MACROPHAGE CELL

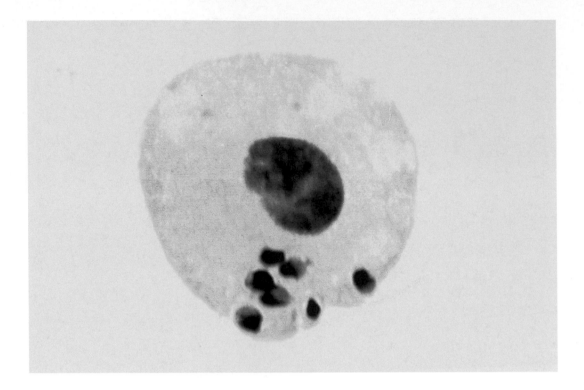

Figure 8.8: Papanicolaou stain (Oil immersion × 5000)

A giant macrophage cell of a diameter of 34.5 microns shows two nuclei superimposed over each other at the center. The upper nucleus has a diameter of 8.8 microns and the lower nucleus has a diameter of 10.2 microns. These nuclei with dense granules are stained blue. The cytoplasm is stained green and appears pale and foamy. At the bottom of the cell few ingested sperm heads with intact acrosomes are seen.

A GIANT BINUCLEATE SPERMIOPHAGE CELL

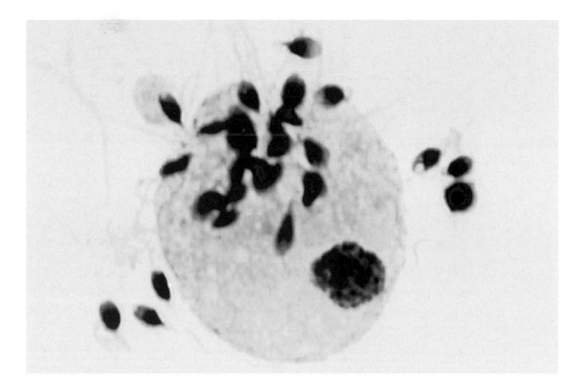

Figure 8.9: Papanicolaou stain (Oil immersion × 5000)

A giant binuclear spermiophage cell measuring 37.2 microns by 31.6 microns has a pair of eccentric overlapping nuclei, situated at five o'clock position. Each of them has a diameter of 8.4 microns. The cell margins are regular. The finely vacuolated foamy cytoplasm shows a group of ingested sperm heads with tails emerging out at the opposite pole of the nuclei.

A BINUCLEATE SPERMIOPHAGE CELL

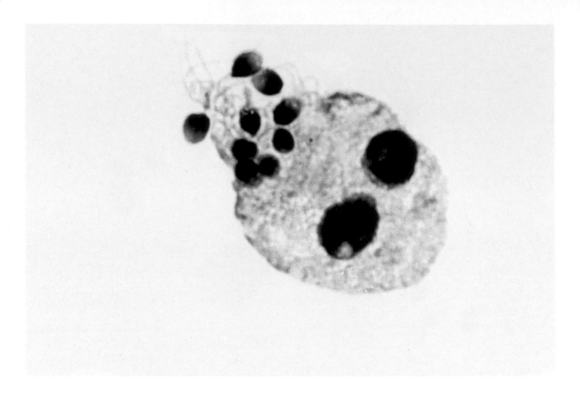

Figure 8.10: Papanicolaou stain (Oil immersion × 5000)

A spermiophage cell, measuring 29.7 microns × 24.2 microns, shows the presence of two opposing nuclei at the center. The upper nucleus has a diameter of 6.8 microns while the lower nucleus has a diameter of 7.2 microns. The nuclei with a dense chromatin are stained deep blue in color. The cell margins, otherwise regular, show a pseudopodium like process at eleven o'clock position with ingested sperm heads. The granular cytoplasm that is stained dense green shows fine vacuolation.

A MULTINUCLEATE MACROPHAGE CELL

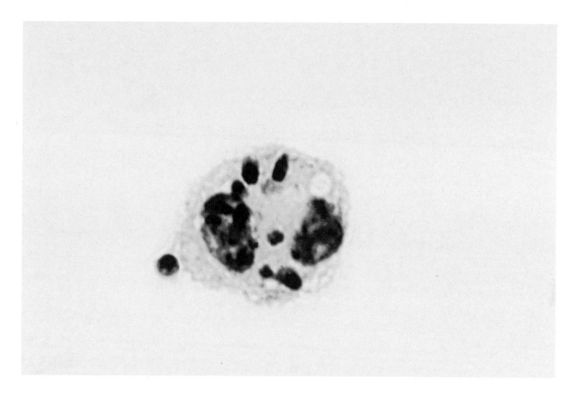

Figure 8.11: Modified Shorr stain (Oil immersion × 5000)

A macrophage cell with irregular margins has four nuclei arranged in two pairs opposing each other. In each pair two oval nuclei are superimposed onto each other. The cytoplasm shows coarse and fine vacuoles. Ingested sperm heads are seen in the intensely stained green cytoplasm.

A DARK TYPE A SPERMATOGONIUM

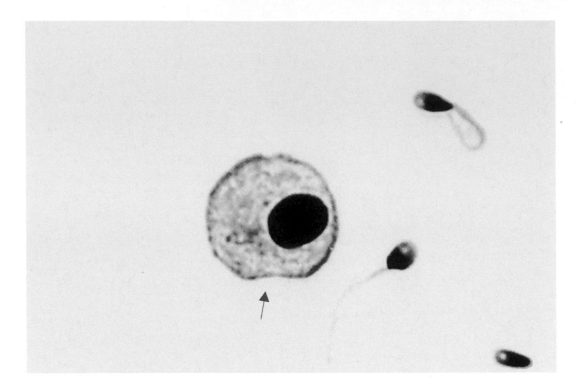

Figure 8.12: Papanicolaou stain (Oil immersion × 5000)

A dark type A spermatogonium measuring 17.38 × 15.66 microns has an eccentric oval nucleus that measures 7.99 × 6.57 microns. One of the cell margin abutting the basement membrane is flattened (arrow). The nuclear details are not seen owing to degenerative changes. The pink cytoplasm shows large pale stained circular area around the nucleus.

The term spermatogonia is derived from the Greek term sperma + gonia (Regeneration).

The primordial germ cells differentiate into Sertoli cells and spermatogonia around the age of six years. The newly formed spermatogonia remain dormant till the onset of puberty.

The term "stem cell " which is often used synonymously has been recently applied to "dormant spermatogonium " which has the potential ability of giving rise to subsequent generations of germ cells.

A DARK TYPE A SPERMATOGONIUM

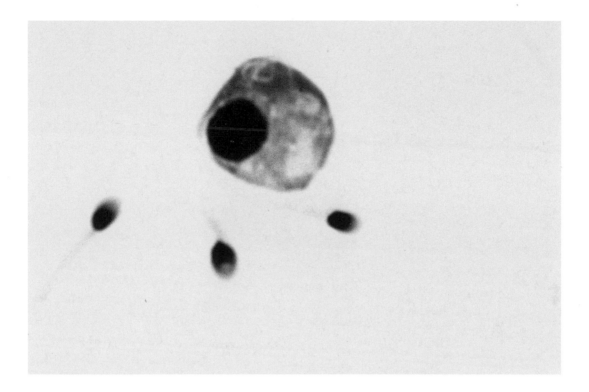

Figure 8.13: Papanicolaou stain (Oil immersion × 5000)

A dark type A spermatogonium measures 18.53 × 17.94 microns. The eccentric nucleus measuring 8.07 × 7.65 microns is darkly stained and shows early signs of degeneration. Two of the cell margins are flattened. The pink stained cytoplasm shows perinuclear pale areas. Spermatogonia are rich in glycogen, the depletion of which results perinuclear hallow areas.

Multinucleate spermatogonia with one to three nuclei may occur (Roosen Runge EC and Barlav FD, 1953).

The first stage of development of spermatogonia is the stage of proliferation. There are seven to eight spermatogonial divisions before spermatogonia mature into primary spermatocytes.

A PRIMARY SPERMATOCYTE

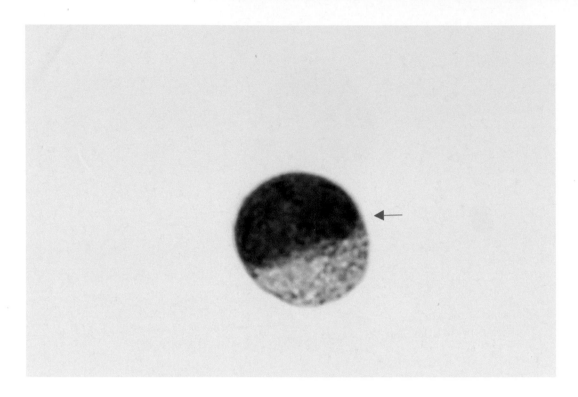

Figure 8.14: Papanicolaou stain (Oil immersion × 5000)

A resting primary spermatocyte measuring 17.57 × 16.45 microns has an eccentric nucleus that measures 16.39 × 11.08 microns. The cytoplasm is stained pink and bluish green.

The primary spermatocytes which are not in the process of division are called "resting spermatocytes". The nuclei of such cells are called "preleptotene nuclei", " interphase nuclei" or "open type nuclei".

The primary spermatocytes are the largest of the germinal cells. The nucleus which is "wooly" is spherical and eccentric. It contains evenly stained chromatin granules, flakes of chromatin and a nucleolus (Arrow). The nuclear membrane is poorly defined. The nucleus has a "wooly" appearance. The chromosomes in this stage remain intact but in somewhat different form (hetrochromosomes) so that small parts of them stain well. These are seen as chromatin granules.

The primary spermatocyte differs from type B spermatogonium which has a well defined nuclear membrane and one of its sides is flattened.

A RESTING PRIMARY SPERMATOCYTE

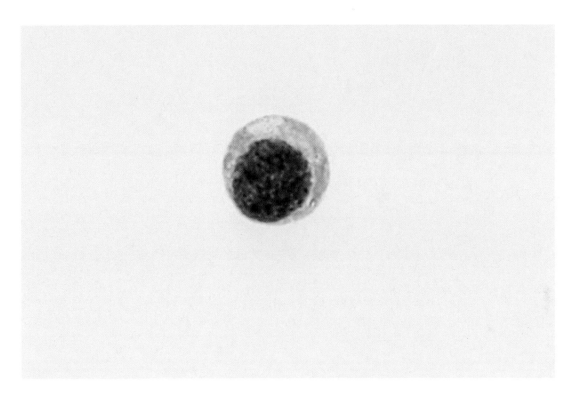

Figure 8.15: Papanicolaou stain (Oil immersion × 5000)

A resting primary spermatocyte measuring 14.08 × 13.5 microns has an eccentric spherical nucleus that measures 11.01 × 9.72 microns. The nucleus with indistinct nuclear membrane shows evenly dispersed chromatin granules. The cytoplasm is stained pink with traces of green.

Most of the enzymes and proteins needed in the subsequent stages of spermiogenesis are synthesized by and stored in the cytoplasm in this cell (Castellani-ceresa L. 1980).

There are two different views regarding the origin of primary spermatocytes. According to some authorities Type B spermatogonia differentiate themselves to produce primary spermatocytes (Roosen-Runge, E.C. 1962). However, according to Ohno (1970) the Type B spermatogonia divide only once to produce primary spermatocytes.

A PRIMARY SPERMATOCYTE—ZYGOTENE STAGE

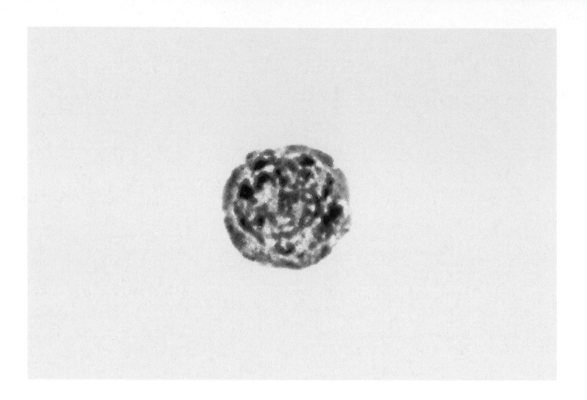

Figure 8.16: Papanicolaou stain (Oil immersion × 5000)

A dividing primary spermatocyte measuring 17.03 × 16.25 microns has a central spherical nucleus that measures 14.09 × 13.20 microns. The network of chromatin is stained deep blue and the cytoplasm is stained pink with traces of green. According to the nuclear changes, the cell is in zygotene stage of meiotic prophase.

In the preceding leptotene stage the chromatin granules had condensed to form fine filaments.

In the zygotene stage the genetically homologous chromosomes are attracted to each other and lie side by side. This process of coupling is called conjugation. Synaptic junction complexes are formed which join the autosomal bivalents. The "X" and "Y" chromosomes must also form bivalents.

So instead of 46 univalent chromosomes 23 conjugated, double or bivalent chromosomes are formed. The chromosomes are stained dark and the synaptic junction complexes are deeply stained. The nuclear membrane disappears and the nucleolus is not visible.

PRIMARY SPERMATOCYTES

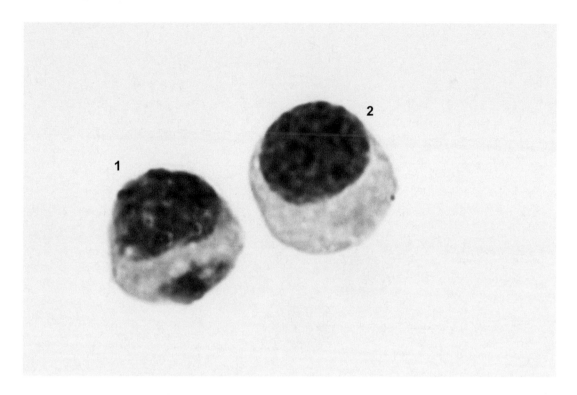

Figure 8.17: Papanicolaou stain (Oil immersion × 5000)

Two primary spermatocytes belonging to 'pachytene stage' of meiotic prophase are illustrated here.

Number 1: A binucleate spermatocyte measuring 17.80 × 14.72 microns has an upper nucleus that measures 10.47 × 10.35 microns. At the lower pole an ill formed second nucleus is seen. The cytoplasm is acidophilic.

Number 2: A mononuclear primary spermatocyte measuring 19.4 × 14.72 microns has a spherical nucleus that measures 14.46 × 12.66 microns. The cytoplasm that is weakly acidophilic is stained pale pink and green and displays fine vacuoles.

In the pachytene stage longitudinal pairing of two autosomal chromosomes is completed and 23 bivalent chromosomes are formed. The bivalent chromosomes become shorter and are coiled around each other. A genetic recombination due to exchange of part of chromatid between homologous chromosomes (crossing over) occurs.

SECONDARY SPERMATOCYTES

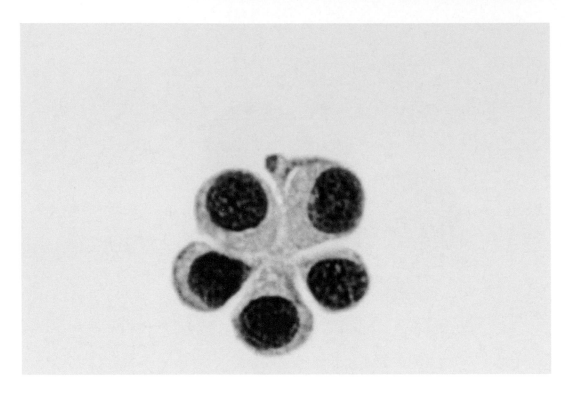

Figure 8.18: Papanicolaou stain (Oil immersion × 5000)

A group of five mononuclear secondary spermatocytes in the resting phase is illustrated here. The spherical eccentric nuclei have evenly distributed granular chromatin.

The average size of the secondary spermatocyte measures 10.25 × 9.05 microns. The average nuclear size measures 7.66 × 6.65 microns.

Secondary spermatocytes have half the size of primary spermatocyte. The life of the secondary spermatocytes is of extremely short duration as they immediately proceed to divide into spermatids.

These cells are diploid in nature and contain 23 chromosomes in the form of diads. Two spermatids originating from a single secondary spermatocyte are haploid in nature and contain 23 chromosomes in the form of monads. One of the spermatids carries "X" chromosome and the other one carries "Y" chromosome.

A MULTINUCLEATE SPERMATID

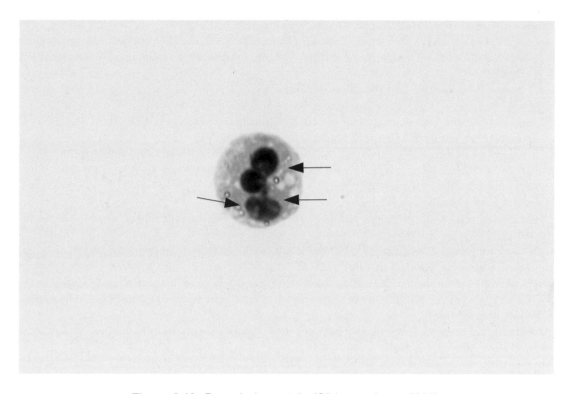

Figure 8.19: Papanicolaou stain (Oil immersion × 5000)

This picture illustrates a spermatid with four nuclei.

A spermatid can have one nucleus or as many as eight nuclei. It is indistinguishable from a secondary spermatocyte save that the former shows the presence of an acrosome. Spermatids are haploid in nature and contain 23 chromosomes in the form of monads.

The nucleus of a spermatid is spherical in nature and has a diameter of 6 microns. In a well stained slide the acrosomal caps of the spermatid nuclei can be identified (Arrows). The nucleus is stained deep blue in the post-acrosomal region and light blue in the acrosomal region. The cytoplasm being acidophilic is stained pink.

In multinucleate spermatids there are often interconnecting bridges.

BIBLIOGRAPHY

1. Anderson DJ. The Effect of Genital Tract Infection and Inflammation on Male Infertility. In : Larry I. Lipshultz and Stuart S. Howards (Eds): Infertility in the Male, 3rd ed. Mosby. St Louis, Missouri 1997.
2. Castellani-Ceresa L. Germ Cells p. 32 In: Hafez ESE. (Ed): Descended and Cryptorchid Testis. Martinis Nijhoff, Boston 1980.
3. EI-Demiry MIM et al. Identifying leukocytes and leukocyte subpopulations in semen using monoclonal antibody probes. Urology 1986;28:492.
4. Eiserman J, Register KD, Stickler RC. The effect of tumor necrosis factor on human sperm motility in vitro. J Androl 1989;10:270.
5. Eliasson R. Seminal plasma, accessory genital glands and infection ; In Cockett ATK, Urry RL. (Eds): Male Infertility workshop, Treatment and Research. Grune & Stratton, Orlando, Fl. 1977.
6. Fowler JE, Jr. Infections of the male genital tract and infertility: a selected review. J Andol 1981;3:121.
7. Gopalkrishnan K, Hinduja I, Kumar IC. Ultrastructure of spermatozoa and non-spermatozoal cells in human semen in genital tract infections. Indian J Med Res 1989;90:175.
8. Jarvi K, Noss MB. Can J. Urol 1994;1(2):25.
9. Krausz C et al. Development of a technique for monitoring the contamination of human semen samples with leukocytes. Fertil Steril 1992;57:1317.
10. Kovalaski, N. de Lamirande, E. and Gagnon, C. Determination of neutrophil concentration in semen by measurement of superoxide radical formation. Fertil Steril 1991;56:809.
11. Leino L, Virkkunen P. An automated chemiluminescence test for diagnosis of leukoctospermia. Int J. Androl 1991;14:271.
12. Matthews GJ, Goldstein M, Henry JM. Nonbacterial pyospermia: a consequence of chlomiphene citrate therapy. Int J. Ferti Menapausal stud 1995;40(4):187.
13. Ohno S. Morphological aspects of meosis and their genetical significance.p.115. In Rosemberg E, Paulsen CA (Eds): The humen testis. Plenum, New York. 1970.
14. Phadke AM. Spermiophage cells in man. Fertil Steril 1975;26:760.
15. Phadke AM. Supravital staining technique for semen Andrologia 1978;10:80.
16. Roosen-Runge EC, Barlav FD. Quantitative studies in human spermatogenesis. Am J Anat 1953;93:143.
17. Roosen-Runge EC. The process of spermatogenesis in mammals. Biol. Rev 1962;37:343.
18. World Health Organization. WHO Laboratory manual for the examination of semen and sperm-ccervical mucus interaction. 4th ed. Cambridge University Press 1999.

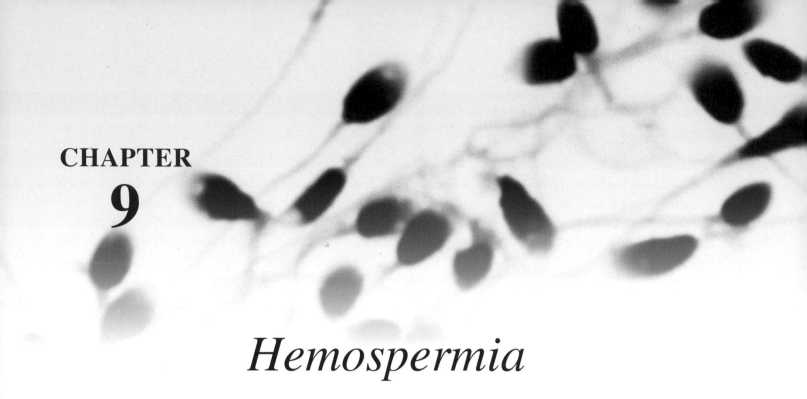

CHAPTER
9

Hemospermia

The occurrence of blood in semen can be a very frightening experience for any male causing great concern and anxiety. His anxiety is compounded when repeated such episodes occur. It seems that this condition was known for centuries and was written about by Hippocrates also.

It is mandatory that every patient complaining of the presence of blood in his semen or noticing a blood stained semen discharge must be thoroughly investigated in order to ascertain the cause.

However, all said and done, the occurrence of a single episode of hemospermia in young adults below the age of 40 years is less likely to be serious. More often than not, hemospermia is such cases tends to disappear spontaneously.

HEMOSPERMIA

The presence of blood in the ejaculate is referred to as hemospermia or hematospermia. It usually presents as an acute fresh blood staining of the ejaculate. It may affect men of any age after puberty, but its peak incidence is in men 30 to 40 years old. Patients having hemospermia may experience repeated episodes.

Hemospermia can be grouped in two categories. The term "Idiopathic" or "Essential" hemospermia is used to describe hemospermia of unknown etiology. The term "Secondary hemospermia" indicates the occurrence of hemospermia due to known etiological factors.

IDIOPATHIC OR ESSENTIAL HEMOSPERMIA

It is commonly observed in young men below the age of 40 years. Most of them have a history of more than one episode occurring at weekly or monthly intervals.

It is essential to ascertain that the bleeding does not originate in the sexual partner. Often sexual habits, such as prolonged abstinence or lack of sex or unusually frequent sex are some of the causative factors. Nelken (1910) and Shropshire (1912), who coined the term "Essential hemospermia," had reported the occurrence of hemospermia in few men indulging in too frequent practice of coitus interruptus.

Though it causes considerable concern for the patients, it is rarely serious, is self-limited and resolves spontaneously with or without treatment.

SECONDARY HEMOSPERMIA

Though semen originates from multiple organs, including testicles, epididymides, vasa deferentia, seminal vesicles and prostate; the bulk of semen comes from seminal vesicles and prostate and pathological lesions in these two organs account for most of the cases of secondary hemospermia.

The etiological factors can be summarized as follows:

TRAUMA

a. Blunt traumatic injuries to testes, perineum and urethra.
b. Following transrectal ultrasound examination (Aus G, Hermanson GG and Hugosson JD et al., 1993).
c. Following transrectal prostate biopsy (Etherington RJ, Clements R and Griffiths GJ et al., 1990; Berger AP, Gozzi C and Steiner H, et al., 2004).
d. Urethral self-instrumentation.

BLOOD IN SEMEN

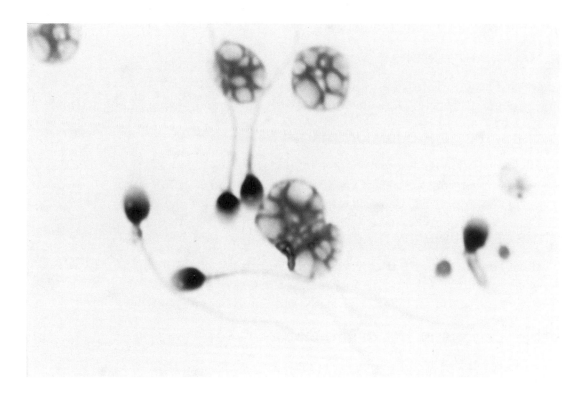

Figure 9.1: Rose Bengal and Toluidine blue stain (Oil immersion × 5000)

The presence of blood in semen is called "Hemospermia" or "Hematospermia" and the semen sample is called "Hemospermic".

Hemospermia is grouped into two categories namely, (1)"Idiopathic" or "Essential" hemospermia and (2) Secondary hemospermia.

In essential hemospermia the bleeding is fresh and hence intact red blood cells are easily identified. The semen specimen is blood stained or brownish. After centrifugation the red blood cells settle down leaving a clear milky supernatant comprising of semen.

In this picture the red blood cells are easily identified. They are mixed with spermatozoa. Note the absence of polymorphonuclear leukocytes.

INFLAMMATION

a. Chronic prostatitis (Papp GK, Kopa Z and Szabo et al., 2003).
b. Acute urethritis. Chlamydial or gonococcal.

BENIGN OR MALIGNANT TUMORS

a. Prostate cancer (Pap GK, Kopa Z and Szabo F et al., 2003).
c. Carcinoma of seminal vesicles (Kawahara M, Matushashi M and Tejima M et al., 1988).

CYSTIC LESIONS IN THE GENITOURINARY TRACT

a. Seminal vesicle cysts (Heller E and Whitesel JA 1963).
b. Congenital cysts of seminal vesicles (Oregid P and Hattleland K 1979).
c. Urethral cysts (Van Poppel H, Vereecken RA and De Greeter P et al., 1983).

CALCULI IN THE GENITOURINARY TRACT

a. Prostate calculi (Etherington RJ, Clements R and Griffith GK et al., 1990).
b. Seminal vesicle calculi (Worischek JH and Para RO 1994).
c. Ejaculatory duct calculi (Iqbal Singh, Sharma N and Singh N et al., 2003).

MISCELLANEOUS LESIONS IN THE GENITOURINARY TRACT

a. Prostate varices (Han MS and Brannigan RE 2004).
b. Prostate telangiectasia (Lamesh RA 1993).
c. Urethral stricture; urethral polyp (Stein AJ, Prioleau PG and Catalona WJ 1980).

SYSTEMIC DISEASES

a. Hypertension (Close CF, Yeo WW and Ramsay LE 1991).
b. Chronic liver disease
c. Amyloidosis
d. Lymphoma (Geoghegan JG and Bonavia I 1990).
e. Bleeding diathesis, e.g. Hemophilia.

INFECTIONS

a. Genitourinary tuberculosis (Yu HH, Wong KK and Lim TK et al., 1977).
b. HIV.
c. Cytomegalovirus {CMV} (Koment RW and Poor PM 1983).
d. Hydatid disease (Halim A and Vaezzadeh K 1980).
e. Schistosomiasis (Lambeli CM and Venkatramaiah NR 1981).
f. Bilharziasis (Elms SS and Patil PS 1987).

Though there are numerous etiological factors responsible for secondary hemospermia, chronic prostatitis, acute urethritis, genitourinary tuberculosis and prostate malignancy in few cases are the commonest causative diseases.

Nonetheless, in every case of hemospermia needs complete investigations including thorough physical examination, checking of blood pressure, direct rectal examination, transrectal ultrasound studies of prostate and seminal vesicles and appropriate laboratory tests to rule out the possible causes of secondary hemospermia.

BIBLIOGRAPHY

1. Aus G, Hermanson GG, Hugosson JD, Pederson KV. Transrectal ultrasound examination of prostate: complications and acceptance by patients. Brit J Urol 1993;7:457.
2. Berger AP, Gozzi C, Steiner H. et al., Complication rate of transrectal ultrasound guided prostate biopsy: a comparison among 3 protocols with 6, 10 and 15 cores. J Urol 2004;171:1478; discussion 1480.
3. Close CF, Yeo WW, Ramsey LE. The association of hemospermia and severe hypertension. Postgrad Med J.1991;67:157.
4. Elm B and Patil PS. Hemospermia: observations in an area of endemic bilharziasis. Br J Urol 1987;60:170.
5. Etherington RJ, Clements R, Griffiths GJ, Peeling WB. Transrectal ultrasound in the investigation of hemospermia. Clin Radiol 1990;41:175.
6. Geoghegan JG, Bonavia I. Hemospermia as a presenting symptom of lymphoma. Br J Urol 1980;66:658.
7. Halim A, Vaezzadeh K. Hydatid disease of genitourinay tract. Br J Urol 1980;52:75.
8. Han M, Brannigan RE, Atenor JA, Roechi KA, Catalona WJ. Association of hemospermia with prostate cancer. J Urol 2004;172:2189.
9. Heller E, Whitesel JA. Seminal vesicle cysts. J Urol 1963;90:305.
10. Iqbal Singh, Sharma N, Singh N, Gangas R. Hematospermia (Ejaculatory duct calculus) - An unusual case. Int J Urol Nephrol 2003;35:517.
11. Kawahara M, Matsuhashi M, Tejima et al. Primary carcinoma of seminal vesicle, Diagnosis assisted by sonography. Urology 1988;32:269.
12. Koment RW, Poor PM. Infection by human cytomegalovirus associated with chronic hemospermia. Urology 1983;22:617.
13. Lambell CM, Venkataramaiah NR. Schistosoma hematobium ova in semen.J Urol 1981;125:603.
14. Lemesh RA. Case report: recurrent hematuria and hematospermia due to prostate telangiectasia in classic von Willebrand's disease. Am J Med Sc. 1993;306:35.
15. Nelken A. Essential hemospermia. J. A. M. A. 1910;55:1200.
16. Oregid P, Hattleland K. Cyst of seminal vesicle associated with ipsilateral renal agenesis. A report of four cases. Scan J Urol Nephrol 1979;13:113.
17. Papp GK, Kopa Z, Szabo F, Erdi E. Aetiology of hemospermia. Andrologia 2003;35:317.
18. Sopshire CW. Essential hemospermia. Am J Dermat and Genito-urin Dis. 1912;16:317.
19. Stein AJ, Prioleau PG, Catalona WJ. Adenomatous polyps of the posterior urethra: a cause for hemospermia. Urology. 1980;124:289.
20. Yu HH, Wong KK, Lim TK, Leong CH. Clinical study of hemospermia. Urology 1977;10:562.
21. Van Poppel H, Vereecken R, De Gector P, Verduyu H. Hematospermia owing to utricular cyst; embryological summary and surgical review. J Urol 1983;129:608.
22. Worischek JH, Para RO. Chronic hematospermia: assessment by transrectal ultrasound. Urology 1994;43:515.

Bacteriospermia

- Meaning of bacteriospermia.
- Scarcity of microbes in semen.
- Categories of bacteriospermia.
  - Infective bacteriospermia.
  - Non-infective bacteriospermia.
  - Fallacious bacteriospermia.
- Common organisms responsible for genitourinay infections.
- Normal vaginal flora.

BACTERIOSPERMIA

MEANING OF BACTERIOSPERMIA

The term bacteriospermia is used to indicate the presence of bacteria in significant numbers in semen.

MICROBES ARE SCARCELY PRESENT IN SEMEN

Bacteria are not normally seen in routine semen smears possibly because of dual reasons. Firstly, muramidase that is secreted by prostate is bacteriostatic and may inhibit bacterial growth. (Rusk J, Tallgreen LG and Alfthan OS et al., 1973). Secondly, the high pH of semen with its high content of lysozymes and Zinc is bactericidal (Mortimer 1994).

SIGNIFICANCE OF BACTERIOSPERMIA

The relevance of bacteriospermia is difficult to gauge due to the variety of situations in which it may or may not be witnessed. It may be of "Infective", "Non-infective" and "Fallacious " type.

INFECTIVE BACTERIOSPERMIA

Patients may complain of local pain and tenderness (as in epididymitis), difficulty in having coital erection and painful ejaculation.

The semen examination may show diminished volume (if seminal vesicles are involved), changes in pH and increased viscosity (if prostate is involved). In prostatic infection the liquification may be affected due to impaired secretion of PSA which is a major enzyme responsible for liquification (Comphaire 1996). Diminished sperm motility may also be observed.

Even in genital tract infections, the pyospermia may or may not be associated with bacteriospermia. The presence of intracellular bacteria in polymorphonuclear leukocytes and macrophages is of uncommon occurrence.

In infective bacteriospermia, only in the acute phase, there is leukocytosis in blood.

Infections of accessory sex glands plays an important role in bacteriospermia. Thus, gonococcal infection may lead to the epididymal obstruction and sperm antibody formation. Similarly chlamydial infection may be responsible for chronic epididymitis resulting in partial obstruction and sperm antibody formation.

Comphaire (1996) has stressed the importance of trivial cystourethritis caused by *Escherichia coli, Streptococcus faecalis,* Klebsiela species and Proteus species in genitourinay infections. According to him it is the most frequent cause of chemical irritation of bladder and urethral mucosa.

Appropriate culture tests and their limitations should be understood. Thus in epididymal obstruction caused by infective organisms, the etiologic agent is not detected by the expressed prostatic fluid culture. Similarly bacterial culture will not detect Chlamydia infection.

In genitourinary infections, the commonest organisms present in semen, in order of their frequency, are listed below.

1. *Ureaplasma urealyticum* 2. *Mycoplasma hominis* 3. *Chlamydia trachomatis* 4. *Escherichia coli* (often found in infections of urinary tract) 5. *Streptococcus faecalis,* 6. *Klebsiella species,* 7. *Proteus species,* 8. *Niesseria gonorrhoeae,* 9. *Trichomonas vaginalis.*

Men who indulge in excessive smoking and those having varicocele are prone to genitourinary infections.

NON-INFECTIVE BACTERIOSPERMIA

The presence of bacteriospermia may not be indicative of any genitourinary infection. Such males are usually asymptomatic. The crucial semen parameters such as pH, volume of the ejaculate, viscosity, sperm motility and the biochemical constituents are not adversely affected.

There is seldom an associated leukocytospermia. Even the bacterial culture may be positive. In such a situation the "bacteriospermia" is referred to as "Non-infective bacteriospermia".

Organisms cultured in semen may not be the cause of pyospermia and may not be contributory factor causing infertility (Cottel E, Harrison RF and McCaffrey MT 2000).

FALLACIOUS BACTERIOSPERMIA

The unclean container used for semen collection, the contamination from the skin, hands and genitalia of the patient are the common sources of contamination which results in misleading bacteriospermia. The presence of adventitious bacteria may owe their origin in patient's urethra and the vagina of his spouse. The vaginal contamination is to be suspected if the semen sample is collected by coital withdrawal.

The normal vaginal bacterial flora after puberty includes Micrococci, Streptococci, Escherichia coli, Lactobacilli, (Döderleins bacilli,) diphtheroids and yeasts (Baur JD, Ackerman PG and Toro, G. 1974).

A simultaneous examination of urine is necessary to rule out any concomitant urinary infection.

The next few pages illustrate some bacteria seen in routine semen smears stained with Rose Bengal and Toluidine blue stain.

COCCI IN PAIRS SEEN IN A SEMEN SMEAR

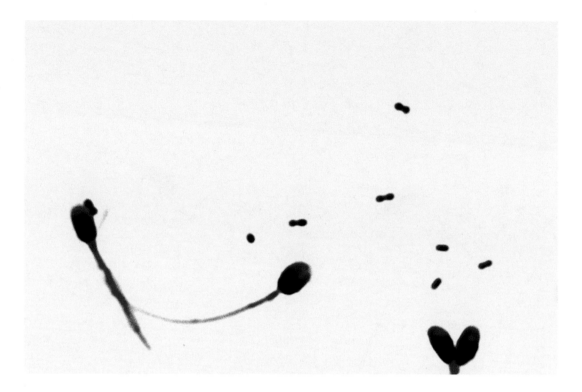

Figure 10.1: Rose Bengal and Toluidine blue stain (Oil immersion × 5000)

This picture illustrates the presence of cocci in pairs, sometimes seen in the routinely stained preparation of semen smears. It is not possible to identify such cocci definitely in absence of Gram's stain. This much can be said that their morphological appearance is suggestive of Streptococci resembling Enterococcus species.

There is absence of polymorphonuclear leukocytes. Hence, one can infer that they could be possibly contaminants.

Hence their presence in a semen smear is indicative of non-infective bacteriospermia, unless confirmed by appropriate culture studies.

COCCI IN PAIRS AND CHAINS IN A SEMEN SMEAR

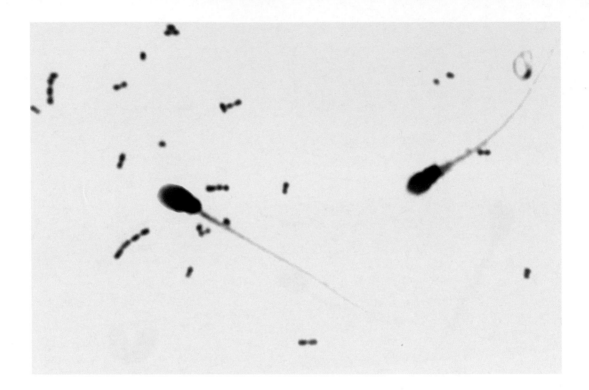

Figure 10.2: Rose Bengal and Toluidine blue stain (Oil immersion × 5000)

This picture illustrates the presence of bacteria, namely, cocci in pairs and chains seen occasionally in semen smears stained for sperm morphology. Presence of bacteria in semen smears is uncommon in the absence of a definite infection. Even in pyospermia bacteria are not always present.

It is not possible to definitely identify these bacteria without a proper staining with Gram's stain. One can, at the best, reasonably guess about their nature from their general morphological appearance. The cocci in pairs and chains, seen in the above picture, have a resemblace to similar cocci of Enterococcus species.

In the absence of associated polymorphonuclear leukocytes response and the appropriate culture studies, it may be assumed that these cocci could be contaminants and a component of non-infective bacteriospermia.

A BUNCH OF SPHERICAL CELLS IN A SEMEN SMEAR

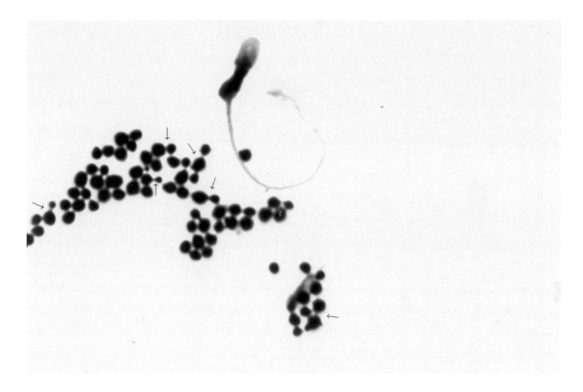

Figure 10.3: Rose Bengal and Toluidine blue stain (Oil immersion × 5000)

The picture shows the presence of a group of spherical cells in a semen smear stained with rose bengal and toluidine blue stain. Morphologically they resemble the "yeast cells." At places budding of the cells can be seen (Arrows). They are stained deep blue with Toluidine blue.

At first glance these cells could be mistaken for cocci arranged in clusters. However, their size is too big for cocci. The budding of the cells leads one to identify them as "yeast cells."

These cells are contaminants from unclean containers used for semen collection, unwashed skin of hands and genitals of the patient. The vaginal contamination, where they are known to be present, can also be a secondary source of contamination.

PRESENCE OF COCCI AND BACILLI IN A SEMEN SMEAR

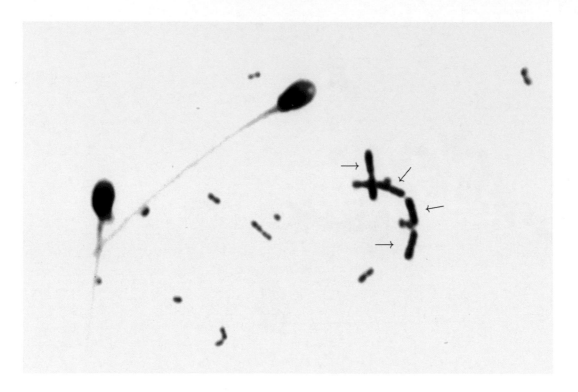

Figure 10.4: Rose Bengal and Toluidine blue stain (Oil immersion × 5000)

The cocci and bacilli seen in this picture are puzzling. The cocci in pairs are morphologically similar to those of Enterococcus species. But what about the thick rod shaped bacilli (Arrows)?

The best guess would be "no guess"! These bacilli are devoid of any spores. One certain thing that can be said is that they are not lactobacilli or Döderleins bacilli because the latter are slender and not so much thick like rods.

A novice may notice a close similarity between the thick rod shaped bacilli depicted above and clostridium perfringens wherein the bacteria are thick, rectangular and may not manifest spores. But a superficial similarity does not offer a valid ground for identification. It will be prudent to describe them as "unidentified thick rod shaped bacilli resembling Bacillus species."

BIBLIOGRAPHY

1. Baur JD, Ackerman PG, Toro G. Methods in microbiology, with reference to methods in virology. In Baur JG, Ackerman PG, Toro G. (Eds): Clinical Laboratory Methods. (8th ed) C. V. Mosby company Saint Louis 1974;p.631.
2. Comphaire FH. Male genital tract infections. In Anibal Acosta and Thinus F. Kruger (Eds): Human spermatozoa in assisted reproduction. The Parthenon Publishing group. New York 1996;P.125.
3. Cottel E, Harrison RF, McCaffrey MT, Waish EM, Barry-Kinsella C. Are seminal fluid microorganisms of significance or merely contaminants? Fertil Steril 2000;74:465.
4. Mortimer D. Semen analysis: Practical Laboratory Andrology. Oxford University Press, New York 1994;p.127.
5. Rusk J, Tallgren LG, Alfthan OS, Johansson CJ. The antibacterial activity of semen and its relation to serum proteins. Scan J Urol Nephrol 1973;7:23.

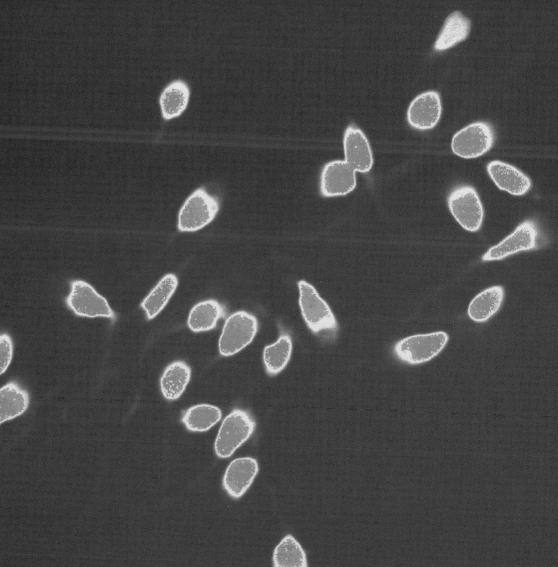

Section 3

Appendices

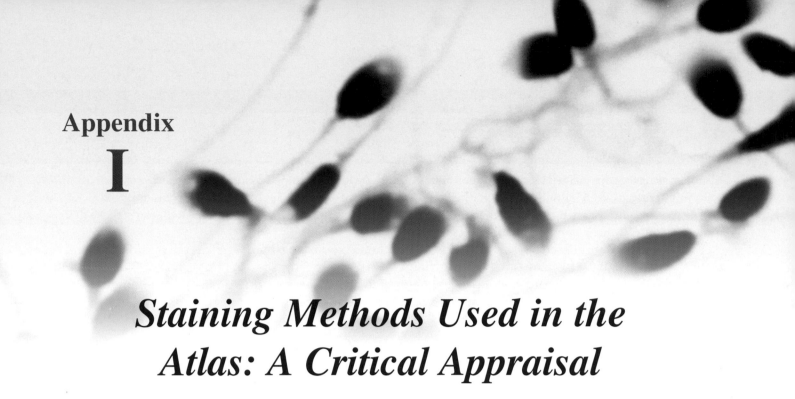

Appendix

I

Staining Methods Used in the Atlas: A Critical Appraisal

STAINING METHODS FOR SPERM VIABILITY:

☐ **Two steps staining techniques**
- Original method of Blom (1950) for bulls
- Method of Dougherty et al., (1975)
- Method of Eliasson (1977, 1981)
- Method described in WHO Manual (1999)

☐ **Methods that use a single stain**
- Method of Eliasson and Triechl (1971)
- Method of Eliasson (1981)
- Method described in WHO Manual (1999)

☐ **One step staining techniques**
- Method of Mortimer (1985, 1994)
- Method of Kvist and Bjömdhal (2002)

SUPRAVITAL STAINING OF CELLULAR ELEMENTS IN SEMEN

- Phadke (1978)

STAINING METHODS FOR SPERM VIABILITY

The assessment of sperm viability constitutes one of the basic steps in semen analysis. It involves identifying non-motile sperms that are viable and non-motile sperms that are dead. The method assumes importance in semen samples with low sperm motility and especially in the diagnosis of necrozoospermia where all the sperms are dead.

The methods for assessment of sperm viability fall in three groups, namely, those that use two stains, those that use a single stain and those that use a combined stain.

All these methods are based on the principle that live spermatozoa have essentially intact cell membranes while the dead spermatozoa have disintegrating cell membranes. Furthermore, the classical observation of Blom (1950) that aqueous solution of eosin is capable of penetrating only the dead sperms (and staining them pink) owing to the structurally defective cell membranes forms the basis of all the staining methods in this group.

METHODS THAT USE TWO STAINS

These methods use 2 steps staining techniques.
  a. **The original method of Blom (1950) for bulls.**

Reagents

- 5% Eosin solution is prepared by dissolving 5 g of Eosin B (C.I. 45400) in 100 ml of distilled water.
- 10% Nigrosin solution is prepared by dissolving 10 g of water soluble Nigrosin (E Merk C.I. 50420) in 100 ml of warm distilled water, allow it to cool and store it in a glass bottle with a stopper after filtering.

Procedure

Place 1 drop of liquefied semen on a clean microscope slide. Add to it 2 drops of Eosin B solution and mix thoroughly for 30 seconds. Add to it 4 drops of Nigrosin stain and mix for 30 seconds. Transfer 1 drop from the semen-eosin-nigrosin mixture to another slide and prepare a smear. Allow the smear to air dry and mount with D.P.X. to store it for future reference.

Examine under oil immersion (1000 x) with a light microscope.

Results

The viable sperms appear white and the dead sperms appear red against a red background.
  a. **Method of Dougherty et al., (1975):** This method is identical to the one described above except that 5% aqueous solution of Eosin Y (C.I. 45380) is used in place of 5% aqueous solution of Eosin B (C.I. 45400) used in Blom's method.
  b. **Method of Eliasson (1977, 1981):** This method uses 1% Eosin Y solution (C.I. 45380) in place of 5% Eosin B used in Blom's method and instead of 4 drops of Nigrosin only 3 drops of Nigrosin are added. The rest of the procedure and results remain unchanged.
  c. **Method given in WHO Manual (1999):** This method is identical to the method described by Eliasson stated above.

METHODS THAT USE A SINGLE STAIN:

These methods use one step staining technique.
  a. **Method of Eliasson and Treichl (1971)**

Reagents

- Eosin Y (C. I. 45380)   0.5 g
- 0.15M phosphate buffer at ph 7.4   100 ml

Procedure

Place 0.1 ml of semen on a glass slide. Add to it 0.1 ml of Eosin Y stain. Mix thoroughly for 1 to 2 minutes, transfer 1 drop from the semen- eosin mixture to another glass slide, prepare a smear and allow it to dry. After incubation of 1 minute examine under oil immersion (1000 x) with a negative phase contrast microscope

Results

The viable sperms appear bluish and the dead sperms appear bright yellow against a dark background.

b. Method of Eliasson (1981)

This method resembles closely to his earlier method (Eliasson & treichl) described above except that the Eosin Y concentration is given as 0.5 to 1%.

c. Method described in the WHO Manual (1999)

Reagents

- Eosin Y (C.I. 45380)   0.5 g
- 0.9% Normal saline   100 ml

Procedure 1

Place 1 drop of semen on a microscope slide, add to it 1 drop of Eosin Y stain, mix thoroughly for 30 seconds and cover with a cover slip. Examine immediately at the magnification of x 400 with a light microscope.

Results

The living spermatozoa are unstained while the dead spermatozoa are stained red.

Procedure 2

Mix 1 drop of semen and 1 drop of Eosin Y stain on a glass microscope slide for 1 minute. Prepare a smear and allow it to dry. Examine the slide under oil immersion (1000 x) with a negative phase contrast microscope.

Results

Live sperms appear black and the dead sperms are stained yellow.

METHODS THAT USE A COMBINED STAIN

Mortimer (1985, 1994) and Kvist and Björndhal (2002) have described the use of a combined stain for assessing sperm viability. These methods use one step staining technique. Hence the unnecessary dilution of semen is avoided.

a. Method described by Mortimer (1985, 1994)

Reagents

Dissolve 0.67 g of Eosin Y (C.I. 45380) in 100 ml of tap water. This solution is heated gently and 10 g of Nigrosin powder (C.I.50420) is added and dissolved before it is brought to boil. The stain is allowed to cool, filtered and stored, in a glass bottle with a stopper, in the refrigerator at 4 degrees C. The stain is warmed to ambient temperature before use.

Procedure

Place 2 drops of semen on a clean microscope slide. Add to it 2 drops of Eosin-Nigrosin stain and mix thoroughly for 30 seconds. Transfer 1 drop from this mixture to another glass side, prepare a smear and allow it to dry. Mount in D.P.X. Examine under oil immersion (1000 x) with a light microscope.

Results

Live sperms appear white while dead sperms show a red coloration or any degree of pink coloration.

b. Method of Kvist and Bjömdhal (2002)

This method is identical to the method of Mortimer described above, except that the stain is prepared in normal saline instead of tap water.

The Eosin-Nigrosin staining methods are often referred to as "Supravital" staining methods. The term "Supravital" used in this context is something of a misnomer given the fact that these methods paradoxically stain the dead spermatozoa and indeed a supravital staining involves staining of a cell in living condition in vitro.

The choice of the method depends on the intentions of the investigator and the laboratory facilities available. If a simultaneous assessment of sperm morphology and the need of the permanent record of the same are the desired objectives, the use of one of the 2 step staining methods or of 1 step combined stain is the natural choice.

Furthermore, the efficacy of the selected method should withstand the scrutiny of its ability to stain the dead sperms in simulated necrozoospermia which can be produced by adding 2 drops of formalin to the semen and waiting for 15 minutes prior to staining.

It will be noticed that in contrast to WHO (1999) method, the one step methods that use the combined stains are incapable of staining all/majority sperms pink or red. As the cardinal use of this method is to diagnose the "true" necrozoospermia, the WHO (1999) method emerges as the method of choice.

SUPRAVITAL STAINING OF CELLULAR ELEMENTS IN SEMEN

Reagents

- Stock solution of neutral red

Neutral red	0.1 g
Normal saline	100 ml

- A working solution is prepared by diluting 1 part of the stock solution with 9 parts of normal saline. Preserve at room temperature (20 to 30 degrees C).

Procedure

One drop of freshly liquefied semen is placed on a clean microscope slide. To it 1 drop of working solution of neutral red is added and mixed thoroughly. One drop of semen-neutral red mixture is transferred to another slide, covered with a coverslip and the edges are sealed with petroleum jelly. Allow the slide to remain at room temperature for 1 to 1½ hours prior to examination.

Results

1. Spermiophage cells: The cytoplasm displays the presence of numerous granules and globules stained bright red. Frequently the cytoplasm is loaded with bright yellow, brown or black pigment material.

2. Spermatogenic cells: The spermatids remain unstained. In the case of spermatocytes two structures are stained with Neutral Red. A) A cluster of granules –called Y granules- near the Golgi region or at extreme end of the cell are stained pink or red. B) A vacuolar structure designated as "Enigmatic body" or "X body" near the nucleus is stained pink or red.

3. Leukocytes: Their coarse cytoplasmic granules are stained orange or bright red.

4. Parasites: A) Trichomonas vaginalis: The digestive vacuoles are stained bright red. B) Balantidium coli (rare occurrence): The digestive vacuoles are stained bright red.

Chief advantage of this method is the easy identification of Spermiophage cells, Leukocytes and Trichomonas. Precursors of spermatozoa are often mistaken for pus cells by less experienced technician and unnecessary antibiotic therapy is given on the basis of such erroneous reporting.

If the author is not to shirk the responsibility of making a candid assessment of his own method, he must concede that the long time required for the staining makes this test impracticable for routine work.

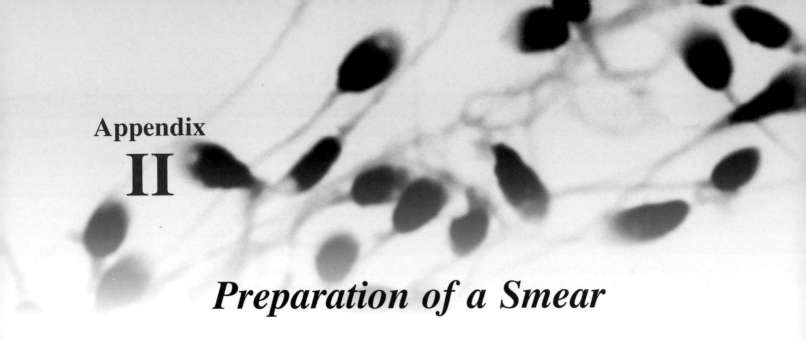

Appendix
II

Preparation of a Smear

The microscope slides should be first washed in a detergent, followed by tap water and wiped with a soft clean cotton cloth or a tissue paper. The coverslips are dipped in ethanol and cleaned with a fiber free tissue paper. With a glass marking pencil write the name of the patient at one end of the slide. Dip the slide in 70% ethanol and cleanse it with soft tissue paper before using.

Always prepare the smears in duplicate so that in case of the smear getting unsatisfactorily stained or disappearing completely (as happens with thick smears) the second reserve slide is available for re-staining.

Remember that the smears are prepared after semen sample is liquefied. To assess this, the semen is aspirated in a dropper and expressed through it. Formation of discrete drops, without string formation indicates liquefaction.

For viscous semen one of the two following methods are used.

1. Place a drop of semen in the middle of a microscope slide. A second slide, face down, is placed on the top of it to allow the drop of semen to spread in between them. Gently pull apart the two slides. Two smears are thus simultaneously prepared.
2. An aliquot of semen (0.5 ml) is diluted with 10 ml of normal saline in graduated centrifuge tube, mixed thoroughly and centrifuged at 800 g for 10 minutes. The supernatant is removed, without disturbing the basal pellet of mucus and debris, and centrifuged again at 800 g for 10 minutes. Remove the supernatant and a drop from the basal sperm suspension is placed on a glass slide, spread it with a dropper to make a smear and allow it to dry.

The practice of repeatedly aspirating the semen in a disposable syringe and expressing it through a 18 or 23 gauge needle several times to reduce the viscosity is to be avoided as it produces distortion of sperm morphology.

For the normal semen samples the following procedure is used.

The semen smear is prepared like a blood smear. The thickness of the smear is controlled by adjusting the inclination of the driving slide. The 'feathering technique', so commonly employed is illustrated on the next page.

METHOD OF PREPARATION OF THIN SMEAR

1 Place one drop of semen at
  one end of a clean slide

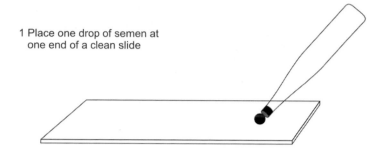

2 Place the driving slide on the top
  of the base slide at an angle of 30
  to 40 degrees

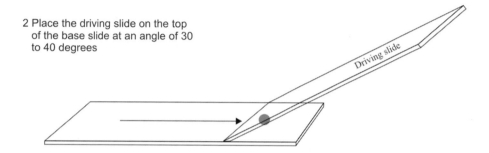

3 Retract the driving slide backward till
  it touches the drop on the base slide.
  The drop will spread along the lower
  end of the driving slide.

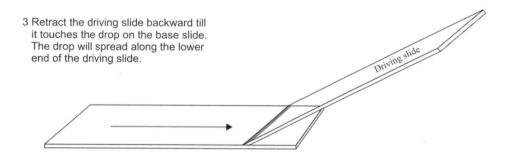

4 Hold firmly the lower slide with
  a finger or against another slide
  placed at right angles and gently
  push the driving slide forwards. A
  thin smear will be obtained

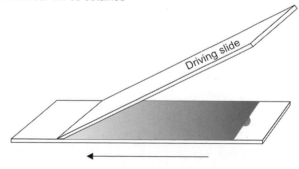

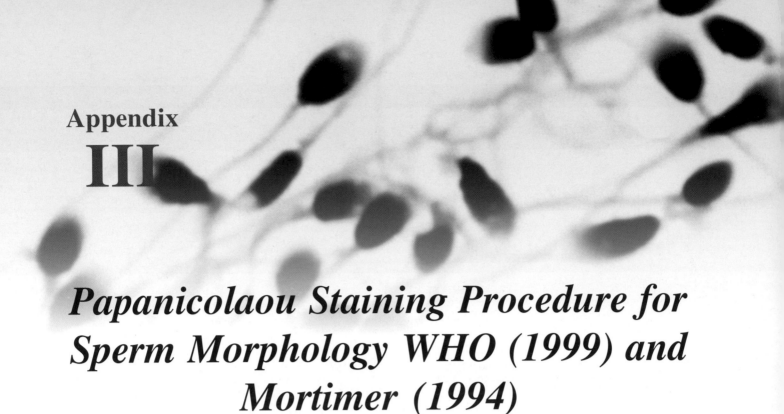

Appendix
III

Papanicolaou Staining Procedure for Sperm Morphology WHO (1999) and Mortimer (1994)

Principal use and features of this stain

The staining of the cell cytoplasm is delicate and transparent because of the high alcoholic content of the stain and the nuclear chromatin is nicely stained. It is an acidophilic/basophilic stain and its chief utility is the differential staining of germinal and non-germinal cells.

Preparation and fixation of the smear

Prepare the smear as described in Appendix II and fix it in ether-alcohol fixative for 5 to 15 minutes.

Reagents

   a. Ether-alcohol fixative: Mix equal parts of 95% ethanol and ether.
   b. Various strengths of alcohol are prepared by volumetric dilution.
   c. Harris hematoxylin: Use commercially available stain. (Papanicolaou solution **1a** Merk) Store at room temperature and filter (Whatman No. 1 filter paper) before use.
   d. OG6: Use commercially available stain.(Papanicolaou solution **2b** Merk)
   e. EA50: Use commercially available stain. (Papanicolaou solution **3b** Merk).
   f. Acid ethanol:

Ethanol 95%	300 ml
Concentrated HCL	2 ml
Distilled water	100 ml

g. Scott solution:

NaHCO$_3$	1.75 g
MgSO$_4$	10 g
Distilled water	500 ml

The two staining procedures, namely the one described in WHO Manual (1999) and the other described by Mortimer (1994) are identical and are considered together.

Staining protocol

• Ethanol 80%	10 dips
• Ethanol 70%	10 dips
• Ethanol 50%	10 dips
• Distilled water	10 dips
• Harris hematoxylin	3 minutes exactly
• Running water (Mortimer 2 dips*)	3-5 minutes
• Acid ethanol	2 dips
• Running water	3-5 minutes
• Scott's solution	4 minutes
• Distilled water	1 dip
• Ethanol 50%	10 dips
• Ethanol 70%	10 dips
• Ethanol 80%	10 dips
• Ethanol 90% (Mortimer 95% *)	10 dips
• Orange G6	2 minutes
• Ethanol 95%	10 dips
• Ethanol 95%	10 dips
• EA-50	5 minutes
• Ethanol 95%	5 dips
• Ethanol 95%	5 dips
• Ethanol 95%	5 dips
• Ethanol 99.5%	2 minutes
• Xylene	1 minute
• Xylene	1 minute
• Xylene	1 minute
• Mount with DPX, allow the mountant to set and examine after 24 hours under oil immersion (X100) objective with a light microscope.	

1 dip corresponds to one second.

The Changes made by Mortimer are given in Parenthesis.

The second slide should be fixed in ether-alcohol fixative for 30 minutes and subsequently air dried and preserved for storage or re-staining if required.

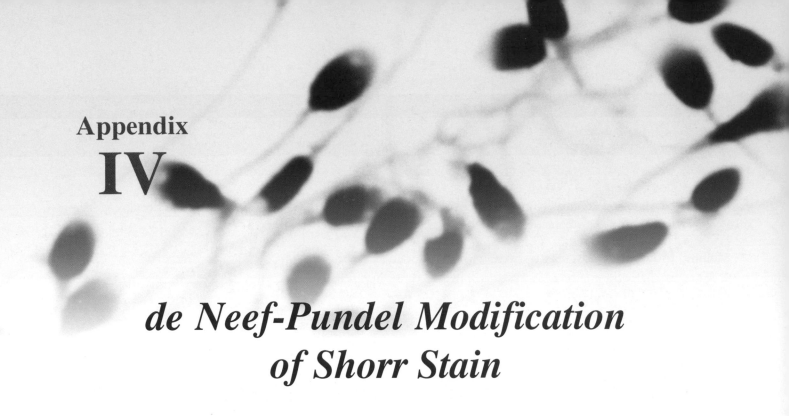

Appendix
IV

de Neef-Pundel Modification of Shorr Stain

Shorr (1941) introduced a single differential stain for vaginal cytology. It is essentially a modification of Masson's stain. It gives only two colors, bright red and greenish blue. However, nuclear details are stained less satisfactorily. Hence it is not commonly used for vaginal cytology.

de Neef-Pundel (See de Neef 1965) modified Shorr's stain to overcome these defects. He has added aniline blue and removed phosphotungstic acid in the original formula of Shorr's stain. His method involves fixation in ether-alcohol and prior staining with hematoxylin.

The author in his experience has found de Neef -Pundel modification of original Shorr's stain more satisfactory for sperm morphology evaluation. This stain is not commercially available and has to be prepared in the laboratory.

Reagents

•	Biebrich scarlet (water soluble)	0.5 g
•	Orange G	0.25 g
•	Fast green FCF	0.075 g
•	Aniline blue (water soluble)	0.04 g
•	Phosphomolybdic acid	0.5 g
•·	Ethanol 50%	100 ml
•·	Glacial acetic acid	1 ml

Dissolve the ingredients in 100 ml of 50% ethanol (warm); allow cooling and then add 1 ml of glacial acetic acid. Filter through Whatman No.1 filter paper and store at room temperature in a tightly capped glass bottle. The prepared stain remains stable for moths together. Filter before use.

The staining procedure is described on the next page.

Staining protocol (Adapted by the author for sperm morphology)

• **Fixation in ether-alcohol for 15 minutes.**	
• Distilled water	10 dips
• Harris hematoxylin	1 minute
• Wash in running tap water	5 minutes
• Ethanol 70%	1 minute
• Ethanol 95%	1 minute
• de Neef stain	1 minute
• Ethanol 70%	5 minutes
• Ethanol 95%	2 minutes
• Ethanol pure	2 minutes
• Ethanol pure	2 minutes
• Xylene	2 minutes
• Xylene	2 minutes
• Xylence	2 minutes.
• Mount with D.P.X.	

Leave the stained slide at least overnight at room temperature for the mountant to set.

Results

The staining characteristics are the same as that of Papanicolaou stain. Thus, the sperm head is stained pale blue in the acrosomal region and dark blue in the post-acrosomal region. The tails are stained blue or pink. The cytoplasmic remnants remaining attached to head, midpiece or tail and the free residual bodies are stained pink.

The cytoplasm of germinal cells is stained in variable pink shades while the nuclei are stained blue or brown. In the case of pus cells and macrophages while the cytoplasm is stained green or bluish green, their nuclei are stained blue. The cytoplasm of epithelial cells is stained blue, pink or orange and the nuclei are stained blue, brown or violet.

de Neef-Pundel's staining method is less cumbersome, less time consuming and simpler than Papanicolaou's staining method and offers equivalent nuclear details.

de NEEF'S MODIFICATION OF SHORR STAIN, FEW ILLUSTRATIVE EXAMPLES

Oil immersion × 5000

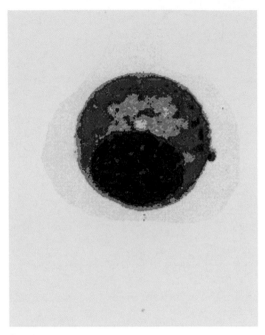

A primary spermatocyte

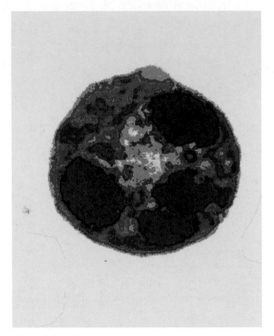

A multinucleate spermatocyte

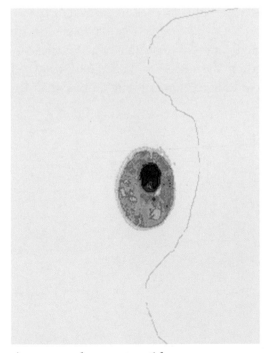

A mononuclear spermatid

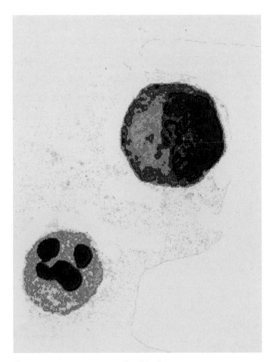

A spermatocyte and a leukocyte

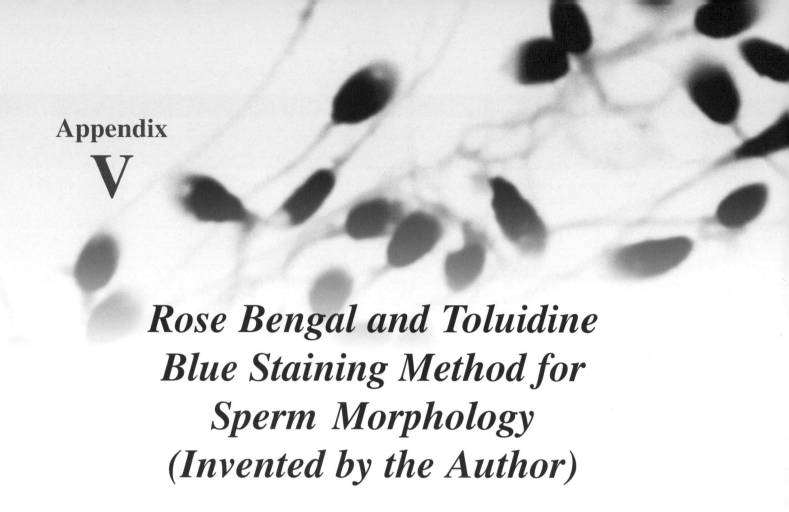

Appendix
V

Rose Bengal and Toluidine Blue Staining Method for Sperm Morphology (Invented by the Author)

This method is invented by the author and is extensively used for illustrating the sperm morphology pictures in this atlas. It is based on the dye replacement technique and is based on the author's original observation that Toluidine Blue stain replaces the nuclear stain from the cellular elements in the semen smear that is previously stained with a specially prepared Rose Bengal stain. This is an inexpensive method, less time consuming and within the reach of a small laboratory and gives excellent details.

Reagents

a. *Rose Bengal 1% stain: Stock solution:* Dissolve 1 g of Rose Bengal stain (C.I. 45440) in 100 ml of warm distilled water and heat it to the boiling point. To the boiling solution add drop by drop and with constant stirring 1 ml of 1% solution of Molybdophosphoric acid (B.D.H. Analar quality $H_3 PO_4 12 MoO_3 24 H_2O$) prepared in distilled water. Allow the stain to cool, make the volume to 100 ml and filter. The filtered stain should have a cherry red color. Store the stain in a bottle with a screw cap.

b. *Toluidine blue stain:* Dissolve 1 g of Sodium Borate in 100 ml of warm distilled water. Add to it and dissolve with constant stirring 1g of Toluidine Blue O stain (C.I. 52040 Merk) and 0.25 g of Lithium carbonate. After cooling filter the stain through filter paper (Whatman No. 1) and store in a glass bottle with a screw cap.

c. Ether Alcohol mixture: Add equal parts of Ether and 95% Ethanol.

d. Phosphate buffers pH 7.4

For the preparation of phosphate buffers please see the next page.

Formula 1:

Solution A:	0.25N Disodium Hydrogen Phosphate:	
	Dissolve 7.101 g of the salt in 200 ml of distilled water	
Solution B:	2 N Hydrochloric acid.	
	Concentrated Hydrochloric acid	2 ml
	Distilled water	9 ml
Final Phosphate Buffer pH 7.4		
Solution A:		200 ml
Solution B:		5 ml

Formula 2:

Solution A:	0.067 M Disodium phosphate solution.	
	Reagent grade anhydrous Na_2HPO_4	9.47 g
	Distilled water	1 liter
Solution B:	0.067 M solution of monopotassium phosphate.	
	Reagent grade KH_2PO_4	9.08 g
	Distilled water	1 liter
Final Phosphate buffer pH 7.		
Solution A		80.6 ml
Solution B		19.4 ml

The solution of the phosphate buffer tends to be cloudy after use and hence is required to be filtered frequently.

The staining protocol

• **Fixation in ether-alcohol for at least 15 minutes.**	
• Ethanol 70%	1 minute
• Ethanol 50%	1 minute
• Tap water	10 dips
• Phosphate buffer pH 7.4 (Use either formula 1 or 2)	1 minute
• Tap water	10 dips
• Rose Bengal 0.25%	20 minutes
• Tap water	10 dips
• Toluidine Blue stain	1 minute
• Tap water	10 dips
• Ethanol 70%	4 dips
• Ethanol 95%	4 dips
• Ethanol	1 minute
• Xylene	2 minutes
• Xylene	2 minutes
• Xylene	2 minutes
• Mount with D.P.X.	

Each dip corresponds to the immersion of the slide of 1 second's duration.

*Working solution of Rose Bengal 0.25% is prepared by four folds dilution of the 'Stock' solution with distilled water.

ROSE BENGAL TOLUIDINE BLUE STAIN (FEW ILLUSTRATIVE EXAMPLES)

Oil immersion × 5000

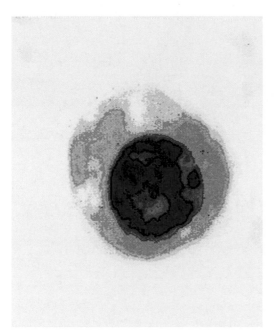

Type A Spermatogonium

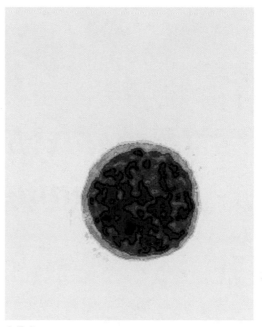

A Primary spermatocyte

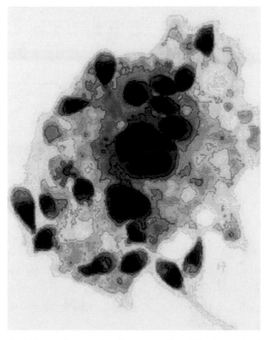

A Giant Spermiophage cell with ingested sperms

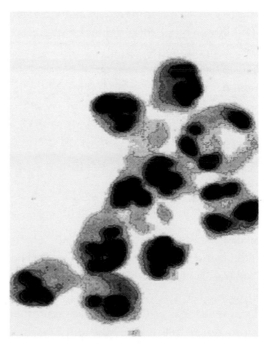

Pus cells in semen

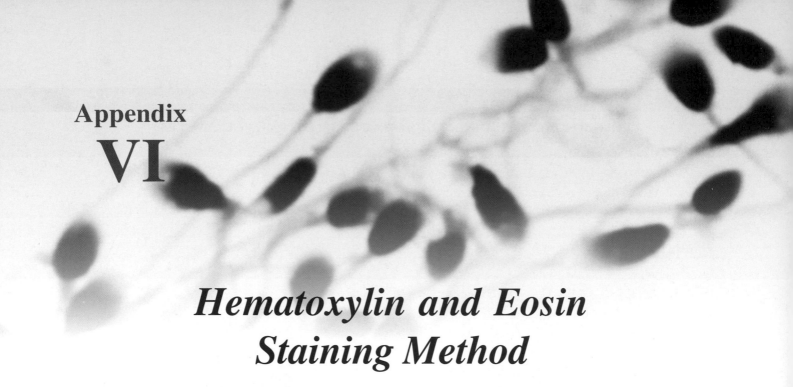

Appendix
VI

Hematoxylin and Eosin Staining Method

Reagents

- Ether-alcohol fixative: Mix equal parts of 95% ethanol and ether.
- Various strengths of ethanol are prepared by volumetric dilution.
- Harris hematoxylin: Use commercially available stain. (Papanicolaou solution **1a** Merk) Store at room temperature and filter (Whatman No. 1 filter paper) before use.
- Eosin Y 0.5% aqueous solution:
Eosin Y (C.I. 45380 BDH)	0.5 g
Distilled water	100 ml
- Acid ethanol
Ethanol 95%	300 ml
Concentrated HCL	2 ml
Distilled water	100 ml
- Scott solution:
$NaHCO_3$	1.75 g
$MgSO_4$	10 g
Distilled water	500 ml

Every pathologist and technician is familiar with H and E stain. However the staining of a semen smear with H and E is not that simple as is believed. The chief difficulty lies in inadequate staining of the tails. Though at present this method is seldom used for sperm morphology, the investigator should familiarize himself with the staining technique because a well stained smear with H and E is better than an ill stained smear stained with Papanicolaou stain.

The staining procedure followed by the author is given on the next page.

Staining protocol followed by the author

- **Fixation in ether-alcohol for 15 minutes.**
- Distilled water — 10 dips
- Ethanol 70% — 1 minute
- Ethanol 50% — 1 minute
- Harris hematoxylin — 6 minutes
- Acid ethanol — 3 dips
- Wash in running tap water — 5 minutes
- Scott solution — 4 minutes
- Eosin Y 0.05% — 10 minutes
- Ethanol 95% — 2 dips
- Ethanol pure — 1 minute
- Xylene — 2 minutes
- Xylene — 2 minutes
- Xylence — 2 minutes.
- Mount with DPX

Leave the stained slide at least overnight at room temperature for the mountant to set.

BIBLIOGRAPHY

1. Blom E. A one-minute live dead sperm stain by means of Eosin-Nigrosin Ferti Steril 1950;1:176.
2. de Neef JC. Clinical Endocrine Cytology. Hoeber Medical Division, Harper & Row, New York 1965.
3. Dougherty KA, Emilson LB, Cockett AT, Urry RL. A comparison of objective measurements of human sperm motility and viability with two live-dead staining techniques. Fertil Steril 1975;26:700.
4. Eliasson R. Supravital staining of human spermatozoa (1977). Fertil Steril 1977;28:1275.
5. Eliasson R. Analysis of semen, In: Burger H, de Krester D (Eds): The Testis. Ravin Press, New York, 1981;p.381.
6. Eliasson R, Treichl ME. Supravital staining of human spermatozoa. Fertil Steril 1971;22:134.
7. Kvist U, Björndahl L. Editorial to the Manual on Basic Semen Analysis. In: Kvist, U. and Björndahl , (Eds): Basic Semen Analysis, ESHRE Monographs, Oxford University Press, Oxford 2002.
8. Mortimer D. The male factor in infertility. Part I: semen analysis, In: Current Problems in Obstetrics, Gynecology and Fertility Volume VII. Year Book Medical Publishers: Chicago, Illinois 1985;p.75.
9. Mortimer D. Practical Laboratory Andrology. Oxford University Press. Oxford, U. K. 1994;p.75.
10. Phadke AM. Neutral Red staining for cellular elements in the semen.Andrologia 1978;10:80.
11. Shorr E. A new technique for staining vaginal smears. Ø A single differential stain. Science 1941;94:545.
12. World Health Organization. WHO Laboratory Manual for examination of Human Semen and Sperm-cervical mucus Interaction. 4th ed. (1999) Cambridge University Press, Cambridge, U.K.

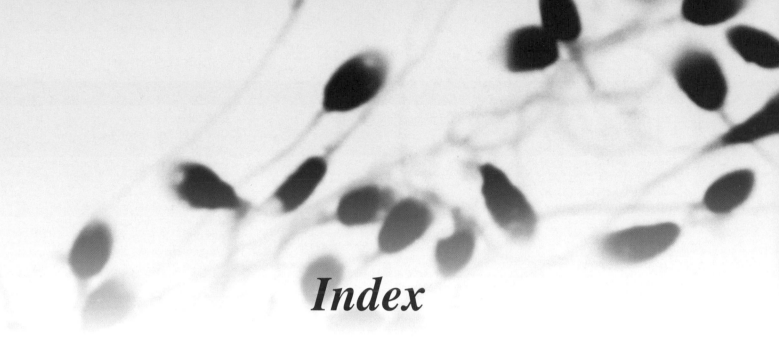

Index